Service Excellence

The Customer Relations Strategy for Health Care

Wendy Leebov, Ed. D.

Authors Choice Press

New York   Lincoln   Shanghai

Service Excellence
The Customer Relations Strategy for Health Care

Authors Choice Press
an imprint of iUniverse, Inc.

For information address:
iUniverse
2021 Pine Lake Road, Suite 100
Lincoln, NE 68512
www.iuniverse.com

Originally published by American Hospital Publishing Inc.

The views in this book are those of the author.

ISBN: 0-595-28367-5

Printed in the United States of America

Contents

Contents

iv

List of Figures

About the Author

Wendy Leebov, Ph.D., is vice-president and general manager of the Einstein Consulting Group, a subsidiary of the Albert Einstein Healthcare Foundation. She has more than 20 years' experience in training and organizational change and currently provides a variety of consulting and training services to health care organizations and businesses nationwide. As codeveloper of HOSPITALity, a comprehensive systems approach to guest relations that has been instituted in more than 100 hospitals, ambulatory care centers, and nursing homes, Dr. Leebov is a nationally recognized expert on hospital customer relations. She has appeared on two teleconferences on customer-oriented management sponsored by the American Hospital Association and has published articles in *Hospital Manager, Personnel Administrator, Health Care Management Review,* and *Hospitals.* Dr. Leebov is editor and publisher of *GRIP: Guest Relations in Practice.* She has a doctorate in human development from Harvard University.

Foreword

I write this foreword for two reasons: first, as Wendy Leebov's friend; and, second, as director of the National Society of Patient Representatives of the American Hospital Association. The National Society of Patient Representatives, and patient representatives across the country, have long espoused the need for health care organizations of all types to become more customer-oriented, to view the needs of their patients—their customers—as their first priority.

Patient representatives began in hospitals to enhance the level of service that patients received, to cut through red tape, and to do for patients what others often did not see as their appropriate role. Today, the role is even more strongly focused in these directions.

Often patient representatives are responsible for the hospital's customer relations or service management program. Certainly this responsibility is consistent with the basic job of the patient representative. However, service is really everyone's responsibility, and this view is critical to the success of any customer relations or service management program.

For such programs to succeed, they must be viewed as cooperative and collaborative, involving everyone in the organization. No longer can organizations move ahead with remodeling, restructuring, and reorganizing, without seeking the input of their patients or employees—their customers.

No one person, or one department, in the hospital can carry the responsibility for customer service programs alone. These programs are multifaceted. They require the entire organization to reexamine itself, from its physical plant and environment to its policies and procedures to its hiring and training practices for employees. We hope this book will help health care organizations to commit the resources necessary to best serve all of their customers.

Alexandra Gekas
Director
National Society of Patient Representatives
 of the American Hospital Association

Preface

☐ The Ripple That Became a Wave

In the few years of its existence in hospitals, customer relations, or guest relations as it was first called, has achieved a history. Today, the burgeoning activity in the customer relations field attests to the importance and strength of the service premise in health care.

Over the last few years, the National Society of Patient Representatives, under the visionary leadership of its executive director Alex Gekas, sponsored teleconferences, workshops, conferences, and symposia to help hospitals strengthen their customer orientation and improve the quality of human relationships with patients and other consumers. Two national newsletters, *GRIP: Guest Relations in Practice* and *National Guest Relations Report*, focus exclusively on hospital customer relations. The American Healthcare Marketing Association, National Society of Hospital Public Relations and Marketing, American Society for Healthcare Education and Training, American Society for Hospital Marketing and Public Relations, Society for Hospital Planning and Marketing, Association of Western Hospitals, Mid-Atlantic Health Congress, Upper Midwest Health Congress, New England Health Assembly, American College of Healthcare Executives, and virtually every other health care association have programs, information, and much activity devoted to the pursuit of service excellence and customer relations.

By the end of 1987, between 60 percent and 70 percent of all hospitals had in place some sort of formal customer relations strategy. According to the National Society of Patient Representatives, more than 48 vendors sell customer relations programs and strategies to hospitals, and many more offer videos and other educational software.

□ A Smorgasbord of Approaches

You name it, and it's been tried.

Some hospitals look to the hospitality industries for their approach because they see that hospitals and hotels share many characteristics: overnight guests; food and housekeeping services; amenities that add to comfort and well-being; and a complex, interlocking system of procedures that have to run smoothly and work for the customer's convenience and satisfaction.

Some hospitals focus on skill building by reinforcing key interpersonal skills, such as techniques for meeting and greeting, anticipating needs, and listening to and coping with complaints. Other facilities focus on motivation, not training, on the premise that people have the skills but have to be motivated to use them. This premise leads to programs aimed at inspiring employee commitment by informing employees about the organization's challenges and getting them committed to doing all they can to ensure their hospital's future.

Some hospitals focus primarily on top management to spearhead the customer relations strategy and integrate it into the organization's culture and everyday management practices. Others say that customer relations is for front-line people, and still others insist it must include every person in the organization, whether or not they interact directly with patients.

Some groups see customer relations programs as finite campaigns with a beginning, middle, and end. Others believe that customer relations must be a vision, a prominent and enduring obsession that drives people's behavior and organizational policy from now to forever.

Some hospitals have entire departments devoted to customer relations. In others, customer relations is only a small part of someone's overall responsibilities.

In short, there are almost as many approaches to customer relations as there are organizations engaged in customer relations activities. And that situation is both a blessing and a curse.

□ A Sophisticated Marketing Tool

With so many different approaches and so much initial razzle-dazzle, the long-term implications of some of the earlier guest relations programs were overlooked. However, this oversight is no longer possible in the competitive environment of health care. Now customer relations and the whole service orientation are increasingly being viewed as a major, primary, lifeblood marketing strategy that can put a health care organization on the map and keep it there in the face of formidable competition and economic forces.

By harnessing the power of an entire work force to excel in customer relations, the forward-moving health care organization of the 1980s and 1990s has a massive sales force devoted to one thing and one thing alone: *the selling of the organization.* And that's what this book is about: how to proceed step-by-step to make your customer relations or service excellence strategy powerful, so powerful, in fact, that it bolsters your employees' service-giving spirit and pride in your organization and also secures your organization's image and economic position in the turbulent years ahead.

□ Experience and Hard Knocks

The cornerstone of this book is the experience and hard knocks suffered by the Einstein Consulting Group in its development of a comprehensive, long-range customer relations strategy, which was named HOSPITALity. In 1982, the Albert Einstein Medical Center in Philadelphia had been experiencing the classic problems of large hospitals in large urban centers in the Northeast. Surrounded by high unemployment, a shrinking tax base, increasing numbers of competitors, and changing reimbursement, Einstein was, and is, faced with the challenge of competing more aggressively in a competitive market.

Marty Goldsmith, then chief of the medical center's Northern Division, thought that employees did not fully recognize their importance to high-quality care and to the image of the hospital. He expressed his belief that employee treatment of patients has a powerful impact on the hospital's image and reputation in the community and, in turn, affects people's decisions about which hospital to use.

After doing considerable homework to get a fix on the customer relations needs and issues at Einstein, we launched an all-out strategy to distinguish ourselves in customer relations. Our objectives were straightforward:

- We wanted to raise the standards of hospitality that every employee extends to every patient, visitor, doctor, and coworker, with the result being greater employee pride in the organization and a level of customer satisfaction that distinguishes Einstein from its competitors.
- We wanted to become known as the high-tech hospital with attentive, warm, wonderful, and compassionate people.

What we had to do was plan a concerted effort to treat patients with special attention. The idea seemed simple enough, but it wasn't. It required motivating the hospital's entire organization, including administrators, managers and supervisors, doctors and nurses, and support personnel from orderlies to maintenance workers. We learned that only a carefully coordinated, comprehensive, hospital-wide strategy could make happen what we wanted to have happen. In designing our HOSPITALity program, we drew on research developments in marketing, organizational change, and corporate culture.

The strategy worked. Our patient satisfaction surveys, image studies, and employee surveys revealed marked improvements in people's perceptions of our employees' treatment of patients and visitors.

☐ Just the Beginning

Over the last few years, together with my colleagues from the Einstein Consulting Group, I have had daily contact with customer relations people nationwide. Their feelings toward customer relations seem to fall into six categories:

- The *powerless,* who are charged with running a program but don't have the resources and administrative support to do it right
- The *stumped,* who have backing but, after launching an initial campaign, don't know what to do next
- The *idea-ists,*who have a wealth of ideas but who have trouble instituting a coherent, long-range strategy
- The *isolated,* who, alone, bear the burden of making customer relations work, because they have few colleagues in their organizations who share their purpose and responsibility
- The *dynamos,* who run successful, flourishing programs but who worry about burning out or running out of steam and ideas
- The *apprehensive,* who haven't begun yet and teeter apprehensively and excitedly on the brink of launching a strategy

If you are in any of these categories, this book should help you by sharing the state of the customer relations art as we at Einstein have come to understand it after years of dips, swings, false starts, and triumphs in our customer relations efforts. To me, customer relations excellence is a sculpture that you have to chip away at bit by bit. My hope is that, as you read, you can learn from our experience, preserve your energy by not reinventing wheels, and build on and surpass our success as you move your organizations forward.

Acknowledgments

I want to thank all the wonderful people who've educated me about the world of customer relations and supported me during the writing of this book:

Many inspirational, incisive, and demanding hospital clients and guest relations directors made this book possible by teaching me the realities and the possibilities.

Katie Buckley, who, in 1982, poured her creative gifts and insights into helping me develop our initial HOSPITALity strategy.

The many people at the Albert Einstein Medical Center, who jumped through hoops to let our group try our approaches before we knew if they would work.

Marty Goldsmith, Mark Levitan, Bob Wise, Holly Tubiash, Bob Goodman, and Paul Stark, who've provided endless support and counsel during the exciting evolution of the Einstein Consulting Group.

Gail Scott for her brilliant, untiring contributions to the customer relations field and for her insights, her Customer Service Matrix model, and her confidence in me.

Our talented, feisty, committed, gifted squad of consultants whose experiences in the field have added brick after brick to our customer relations fortress: Marsha Kurman, Allan Geller, Jack Fein, Gail Murphy, Susan Afrait, and Paul Murphy.

Acknowledgments

Linda Schroeder, Marjorie Ziff-Levine, Michelle Collins, Sandy Tafler, Joan Theetge, George Frascatore, Silvia Bloise, Virginia Yeager, Jeanne Joseph, Jana Griffith, Bill Johnson, Roz Shaw, and so many others too numerous to mention who have helped, typed, researched, stapled, covered for me, and kept me laughing so I could churn out the words.

Sandy Weiss from American Hospital Publishing, Inc., who encouraged me and polished my prose.

My parents and sister for their blind confidence.

Liz and Nikki for unending support.

My grandmother whose last days made me want to make all hospitals better for everyone's loved ones.

Heartfelt thanks to you all.

□Part One

An Organizationwide Strategy

BWATP or What's It All About?

Real Story No. 1: The Knee
We are on attending rounds with the usual group: attending, senior resident, junior residents, and medical students. There are eight of us. Today we will learn how to examine the knee properly.

The door is open. The room is ordinary institutional yellow, a stained curtain between beds. We enter in proper order behind our attending physician.

The knee is attached to a woman, perhaps 35 years old, dressed in her robe and nightgown. The attending physician asks the usual questions as he places his hand on the knee: "This knee bothers you?"

All eyes are on the knee; no one meets her eyes as she answers. The maneuvers begin—abduction, adduction, flexion, extension, rotation. She continues to tell her story, furtively pushing her clothing between her legs. Her endeavors are hopeless, for the full range of knee motion must be demonstrated. The door is open. Her embarrassment and helplessness are evident.

More maneuvers and a discussion of knee pathology ensue. She asks a question. No one notices.

More maneuvers. The door is open.

Now the uninvolved knee is examined: abduction, adduction, flexion, extension, rotation.

She gives up.

The door is open.

Now a discussion of surgical technique. Now review the knee examination. We file out through the open door.

She pulls the sheet up around her waist. She is irrelevant.

□ □ □

Real Story No. 2: Treat with Respect

Rebecca Roberts, a long-term victim of rheumatoid arthritis, had already had multiple hospitalizations for major reconstructive surgery, including hip and knee joint replacements and months of rehabilitation. She had faced each impending surgery with courage, strength, and determination to combat an erratic and disabling disease.

Then Rebecca was faced with another surgery. A hip replacement had to be totally redone, and the doctors warned that the prosthesis might not adhere. If this procedure failed, Rebecca could face lifetime confinement to a wheelchair.

Sensing depression and anxiety that was unlike her, her friend Mary C. Pappas sat down with her to talk. Rebecca said she understood the prospects and risks of surgery. She had faced them before and she would face them again. The gravity of the prognosis was not what upset her. What upset her was making one more hospital employee understand that she is an intelligent, capable, thoughtful person, who is able to make her own health decisions and who deserves respectful treatment. She whispered tearfully, "I can't listen to one more patronizing, demeaning statement from an employee. I just don't have the energy for it anymore."

Mary felt helpless. She tried to think of something to do, some gift that would combat the depersonalization and humiliation Rebecca knew she faced. Mary decided to make a sign. Knowing how strict hospital signage policies are, she had it typeset in Helvetica Medium by a professional sign company and in the hospital's approved color format to conform to hospital policy.

On the morning of the surgery, with the cumbersome two-foot by three-foot sign in hand, Mary entered Rebecca's room. With her parents and husband surrounding her, the mood was one of quiet resolution. Mary silently placed the sign on the wall opposite her bed and gave her these instructions: "When you return from surgery, during your stay, your recuperation, and your rehabilitation, when anyone gives you any difficulty, just point. Don't talk; just point." The sign said:

ATTENTION: MEDICAL STAFF AND EMPLOYEES
PATIENT: Rebecca Roberts
HISTORY: Intelligent creative artist
             Talented published writer
             Poet
             Magnificent human being
             X rays denote grossly positive sense of humor
ALLERGIES: "WARNING!"
             Severe allergic reaction to:
             • depersonalization
             • patronization
             ANTIDOTE: Treat with massive doses of
                       intelligence, sensitivity, and
                       excellent medical care p.r.n.
PROGNOSIS: STROLLING SUMMER SUNSETS

Rebecca's stay was better this time. Physicians and employees read the sign, looked at the floor, and then treated Rebecca differently, with the respect she deserved. Also, word traveled fast. Dozens of other patients and their families came to see the sign and to ask how they could get one.

(Reprinted with permission from Mary C. Pappas, copyright 1987)

□ □ □

Real Story No. 3: BWATP

At an educational session in Phoenix on patient-centered medicine that was sponsored by Grantmakers in Health, the attending executives, whose foundations fund health care projects, began their discussion with a focus on patient needs. Soon, the discussion turned to economics.

Suddenly, Travis Cross, a trustee of the Fred Meyer Charitable Trust in Portland, Oregon, pulled a beautiful brass plaque out of his briefcase and set it in front of him. The plaque had only the initials BWATP on it.

Mr. Cross was asked what BWATP meant. He flipped over the fancy brass plaque, and it read *But What about the Patient?*

Mr. Cross had this plaque made for use in his many meetings with grants people, administrators, accountants, physicians, and others who, in his opinion, quickly lose sight of the patient in their labored decision making. He says he needs something to refocus people when they forget what business they're in.

□ □ □

☐ That Magic Touch of Humanism

These examples, and countless others like them, show the importance of that magic touch of humanism. People who need hospitals are sick, vulnerable, and worried. They've seen better days. For an endless variety of understandable reasons, hospitals seem to have forgotten about the patient, and they shouldn't. If hospital professionals were patients, they wouldn't settle for less than the most humanistic treatment. If their loved ones were in those beds, they would fight to the death for the best the hospital could offer.

Everyone in a hospital, no matter what that person's job is, should be guided by what has been said is a physician's job: "a doctor's job is to cure sometimes, relieve often, but comfort always." That philosophy has been at the heart of the healing arts since the beginning of recorded history.

For all the recent turmoil in the health care and medical professions, one fact remains unmistakably clear and irrefutable: medicine and health care are humanistic activities. No matter how much high technology, how many machines and microchips, are involved in the diagnostic process, the backbone of health care is its "laying on of hands." People's experiences at the hands of a doctor, nurse, or any other member of the health care profession are intensely personal, intensely human. A person in a hospital needs that human touch, that caring and compassion and love that in itself can do miracles even when technical and professional skills can do nothing.

People live in a highly technical, often impersonal world. Machines have taken over to an extent that even H. G. Wells did not conceive. Hospitals are caught in a crunch. On the one hand, a health care institution must provide its users with state-of-the-art diagnostic and procedural services. That's what the public expects. On the other hand, people expect the tender loving care that has, since Florence Nightingale, been part of the care giving culture.

The more high-tech equipment and technology in a facility, the more frustration and alienation for both health care providers and their patients. Technicians stand behind computer screens; printouts offer diagnostic information; and a complex series of buzzers, beepers, and other "new-fangled" devices stand between the patient and the provider. Because hospitals must provide the best possible medical care that contemporary technology makes available, high tech became king, and high touch took on lesser importance in the preservation of human health and human life.

In the mid-1980s, this picture began to change. Because of massive fiscal and market pressures, hospitals started scrambling for patients. But they all offered the same things—the high-tech miracles, digital diagnostics, and all the other procedures of a machine age. Hospitals had to look for a way to distinguish themselves, to locate a factor that would attract and secure a loyal following of patients and physicians and solidify a wavering census. The time was right for the appearance of innovative options for service. Only the fittest and feistiest would survive. Anything that is legal, ethical, and profitable will probably be tried. One of the ideas that was tried was customer relations.

How ironic that the care and love that had traditionally epitomized health care needed a strong, external market-driven motive to reassert itself and gain its rightful place. Because of the severe frustration levels experienced by both patients and care givers, the climate became ripe for attention to customer relations in the hope of reducing these tensions. Hospital leaders wanted to build a new image of hospitals as a service-oriented business intent on achieving excellence. Their strategy was built on the premise that the quality of caring and warmth and the comforts and personal attention offered by service-oriented people can go a long way in making both patients and staff feel human in a high-tech setting and to make patients feel at home, where they wish they were in the first place.

☐ Service, Service, Service

The health care consumer is more sophisticated, demanding, and educated than ever before. This new consumer has alternatives, a veritable smorgasbord of hospitals, outpatient services, holistic health centers, and the like. If your organization is going to be among the survivors, consumers must choose your organization when they shop among the smorgasbord of alternatives.

What is the most influential factor in consumer choice? The answer is *service*. After all, consumers know how to evaluate service, even though they may not know how to evaluate health care.

Just look at the range of options available for making a long-distance phone call, taking a trip, purchasing a computer, or eating Italian food. The single factor by which consumers make their choice, assuming price and availability are similar, is *service*.

The same goes for health care. With all technical variables being equal, consumers go for health care to the organization that provides them with service they can see and experience rather than with medical and technical services they can't see or judge adequately.

People who have doctors may take their doctor's advice about which health facility to use. However, people are taking their doctor's advice less than before. They are also more likely than ever before to shop around for doctors who refer them to facilities they respect, ones with a reputation not only for medical excellence, but also for excellent service and caring personnel. People use the same criteria to evaluate health care facilities that they use to evaluate other service organizations. At a National Healthcare Marketing Symposium held in 1985 in Kansas City, John Cottillion, vice-president of planning and marketing for South Community Hospital in Oklahoma City, summarized why customers don't go back to an organization:

- 1 percent die
- 3 percent move away
- 5 percent seek alternatives or substitutes
- 9 percent go to the competition
- 14 percent are dissatisfied with the product
- 68 percent are upset over bad employee attitudes that resulted in mistreatment of the customer

An advertisement from United Technologies puts it well: "We no longer live in an era of caveat emptor; this is the era of caveat vendor. The lesson is clear: the vendor who fails to provide excellent service loses to a competitor who does—a competitor who has listened better, heard better, and had the courage to act even when such action necessitated change."

☐ Bad News Has Wings

> The most important thing to know about intangible products is that the customer usually doesn't know what he's getting until he doesn't. Only when he doesn't get what he bargained for does he become aware of what he bargained for. Only on dissatisfaction does he dwell.
> Satisfaction is, as it should be, mute. Its prior presence is affirmed only by its subsequent absence.
>
> —Theodore Levitt in *The Marketing Imagination* (New York City: Free Press, 1983, p. 105)

According to the TARP: Technical Assistance Research Project in Washington, DC, if you satisfy 1 customer, they tell 4 others. If they are steamed, they tell 11. Thus, when you annoy one customer, you have to satisfy 3 just to stay even.

The fact is that health care is a hot topic. Everybody has something to say about it, and people listen to what's being said. Frank J. Weaver, director of public affairs and corporate development for the Cleveland

Clinic Foundation (CCF) in Ohio, reports that a study done in 1986 of new patients at CCF shows that the interpersonal media, and not television and other mass media, influence consumer choice among specialty health care providers (figure 1-1).

Clearly, in a competitive environment, health care organizations have a stake in making sure the grapevine draws people to them, instead of turning them away to their competitors. Consider the 10-10-10 principle used in business:

> It takes $10,000 to get a customer.
> It takes 10 seconds to lose one.
> It takes 10 years for the problem to go away.

Figure 1-1. Sources That Influence Consumer Choices of Health Care Provider

Source	Percent
Interpersonal media	88.2
Family physician	34.1
Family member	24.7
Friends	14.3
Former patients	10.5
Employees	11.0
Other	4.6

©1986 by the Division of Public Affairs, the Cleveland Clinic Foundation. Reprinted with permission.

☐ The Hospital's Tarnished Image

> Reputation, reputation, reputation! O! I have lost my reputation. I have lost the immortal part of myself, and what remains is bestial.
>
> —Shakespeare, Othello, II, iii

The public no longer idolizes the health care organization or the care giver. Media coverage and people's own experiences have pushed health care off its former pedestal of respect and destined it to a life of scrutiny.

In the June 30, 1986, issue of *Newsweek*, Meg Greenfield wrote that the hospital experience is "a maddening combination of individual excellence and systematic incompetence, the one tirelessly and heroically saving life and limb, the other forever putting both at mindless risk." She goes on to say that hospitals "are presided over and manned by human beings and that they are at a minimum fallible because the good guys and good instincts don't always prevail. . . . They and their technological equipment operate against a background of remorseless human shortcoming, bureaucratic inefficiency and indifference. That, not some need to understand the exotic equipment or science, is the problem. What is required is a fundamental, painstaking re-education process on the part of the whole institution—a relearning of attentiveness, individual accountabililty, care."

With the media emphasizing the skyrocketing cost of health care, the public increasingly sees hospitals as money-hungry businesses that have lost their charitable roots and concern for human welfare. The public brings this mind set with them when they seek care or visit friends or relatives in hospitals. Hospital employees have to recognize and not be infuriated by negative stereotypes and low expectations. Instead, they must create a new reality, one that shows the hospital's continued concern for helping people as well as its need to pay its bills and support itself.

□ The Only Constant Is Change

> We don't know where we're going, but,
> quite clearly, we're getting there awfully fast.

Hospitals have sprinted through a period of rapid growth, followed now by a period of traumatic cutbacks, downsizing, and change, change, change. Things aren't as they were. Most people who entered health care because it was "secure" are now overwhelmed with anxiety and the disappointment of broken promises at the same time that they are being pushed to work even harder.

An instinctive reaction to change for many of the country's hospitals has been to develop marketing strategies, hire marketing experts, and build a marketing structure to stave off the negative forces of the marketplace. These marketing experts pinpointed similar marketing problems and shared them with their hospital clients:

- *Lack of differentiation.* Many hospitals serve the same market and have essentially the same product and service mix. Most offer obstetrics, pediatrics, a women's center, an on-site pharmacy, good surgical staff, an outstanding cardiologist, and the requisite cafeteria and coffee shop.
- *Competition for referral business.* Many hospitals compete heavily

for physician referrals to their internal specialists. In so doing, most offer the same incentives, such as easy parking and garage access to the hospital, patients located in rooms as close to one another as possible; staff lounge with telephones, coffee, sodas, and other amenities; and an ongoing mail campaign to keep referring physicians updated on hospital services.

- *Diversification.*Hospitals are urged by their consultants to diversify in an attempt to shore up eroding revenues. Hospitals consider similar demographic and market analyses and similar diversification options. Most hospital presidents hire in-house public relations and marketing staff. Most hospitals begin to consider acquisition of nursing homes and a variety of joint ventures from urgicenters to medical office buildings to linen services.

- *Advertising and public relations.* Many hospitals allocate large sums to advertising, and soon ads for similar services from these institutions begin to appear in the marketplace. The hospitals use billboard ads, full-page display ads in the daily papers and Sunday supplements, commercials on radio and television, massive direct-mail efforts, and every other type of advertising and promotion available. The ads make big promises to the consumer.

Despite impressive marketing efforts, some hospitals met with disappointing results. Others became worried that they couldn't keep their ambitious promises once the customer opts for service in their institution. The patient-consumer can't really differentiate between the hospitals and their services. Referring physicians remained unimpressed with fancy sofas and hot coffee when it took their patients four hours of tedious waiting before getting a room assignment. The only satisfaction came to the local media, which suddenly found itself with a new, large, and essentially unsophisticated advertiser: the local hospital. Also, most marketing efforts have not increased admissions, improved the bottom line, stemmed expensive turnover problems among nurses, or improved morale and services.

Change has caused the future of the health care industry to be uncertain, and this uncertainty generates fear. Mergers and acquisitions, hospital closings, intense competition, difficult and demanding consumers—all these elements create an atmosphere of confusion and tension.

As a result, most health care organizations acknowledge, or are beginning to acknowledge, that they must become increasingly customer driven and must consciously and conscientiously strive for service excellence. They must un-quo the status. Marketing surveys, advertising campaigns, targeted product lines, and services for segmented and specialized market groups are rocking health care

11

institutions straight into the service economy.

Machines do not a hospital make. To remain successful in a competitive health care market, your organization must outperform its competitors on the human dimension.

The challenge is to provide high-quality care and caring in the face of extreme pressure. The reputation of your organization and the self-esteem of your employees rest on making your patients' needs the hospital's paramount responsibility and not letting the hospital become either self-absorbed with anxiety and disillusionment or obsessed with the bottom line. Your hospital must back up clinically excellent health care with a concerted effort to satisfy your customers and bolster the caring attitude, job satisfaction, and self-esteem of all of your employees. That's what customer relations is all about.

□ **Chapter 2**

Internal Marketing: The Business Side

The Rude Receptionist Scenario
In the Sunday paper, Ms. Brown saw an ad for an obstetrical program
sponsored by a local hospital. The double-page spread, which cost the
hospital $24,000, was promoting a packaged birthing program for
$395. The package included a new birthing room, which accommo-
dates the spouse; a special bed that would serve for both labor and
delivery; Laura Ashley prints on the furniture and drapes; a welcoming rose, and other delights reminiscent of a luxury resort.

Here's what happened when Ms. Brown, who is expecting her
first baby in seven months, called to find out more about the facility,
the package, the physicians, and any extra charges. The phone rang 32
times before someone answered, and then before Ms. Brown could say
a word, she was put on hold. She was kept waiting for five minutes,
during which time the receptionist not once came back on the line to
tell her that someone would be with her shortly. When Ms. Brown was
finally able to voice her request for more information, she was
shunted from department to department, placed on hold several more
times, and finally told that someone would call her back. Days
passed, and she received no follow-up call.

Seven months later, Ms. Brown gave birth to a beautiful, 8-pound
girl at another hospital.

□ □ □

The X-Ray Shuffle: The Oldest Dance-Step in Health Care
Mr. Jones is 67 years old and has been admitted to his local hospital for

13

tests, including X rays. On the second day of his stay, Mr. Jones is placed on a gurney by an attendant with cold hands and wheeled down public corridors crowded with visitors, children, and staff members. From the elevator, where he is stared at in uncomfortable silence by everyone who gets on and where he has only the ceiling to look at, he is pushed down several corridors and left outside the x-ray department. He is not told how long he must wait nor is he asked if he is comfortable, hot, cold, bored, tired, or thirsty or if he needs to void his bladder. Again he has only the ceiling to look at and his own fearfulness for company.

People in assorted hospital uniforms rush by, but no one stops to chat for a moment or to ask if they can do anything for this frightened old man. An hour passes, and then another. Finally, he is unceremoniously taken back to his room and told that his X rays will be taken later. He is not told why he was kept waiting or when the tests will be made. Three hours later, the procedure is repeated.

□   □   □

The "I'm Lost" Scenario
A newly arrived immigrant family comes to the hospital to visit an ailing relative. The family speaks virtually no English. They check in at the main desk to ask where the room is located, and the receptionist waves them toward several banks of elevators. They get on the wrong elevator and wander the halls, obviously looking lost. People rush past. An orderly bumps into them with a tray of instruments and mutters a rude word under his breath. A nurse, irritated by the interruption, tells them they're on the wrong floor. Confused and embarrassed, they wander around feeling out of place and unwelcome.

□   □   □

The Broken TV Scenario
Mrs. Green has been in and out of hospitals with a variety of chronic ailments for several years. Her poor health and the economic burden it has placed on her and her family have made her cranky and irritable most of the time. In fact, the nurses rarely pay attention to her anymore because she always finds fault with everything.

One day, she turns on her hospital-leased TV only to find, just as her favorite program is about to begin, that it is out of order. She calls the nurse and reports the fact that her TV isn't functioning. The nurse says she'll take care of it. Mrs. Green waits a few hours and then calls again. By this time, the shift has changed, and another nurse tells her she'll check on it. More time passes.

By the time the TV set is repaired, Mrs. Green has waited three days, talked to a dozen people, and is crankier than ever. Her mood just reinforces the staff's view of her, and she receives even less care and attention. What makes the situation so much worse is that Mrs. Green has an eye ailment, and so she cannot read or do any close work. Television is her company.

☐   ☐   ☐

The Cold Dinner Tray Scenario
The dinner tray arrives 40 minutes late. Not only is the order incomplete, but the food is stone cold. The patient is annoyed, asks for it to be changed, and is told that the kitchen is closed.

☐   ☐   ☐

The Loss-of-Dignity Scenario
The patient in room 234 is bedridden and can't use the bathroom. It seems that every time she's on a bedpan, a parade of nurses, attendants, and assorted doctors arrives in her room. None of them ever knocks or asks permission to come into what is essentially her bedroom. They seem unaware of the importance of giving her privacy or time to cover herself up to maintain her modesty and dignity.

☐   ☐   ☐

☐ The Market Loss

These anecdotes are not fiction. They happen in hospitals that spend thousands of dollars on flashy ads and glossy brochures but keep rude receptionists, make patients wait for X rays without explanation, deliver incorrect and poorly prepared food, don't allow even the most basic privacy, and don't maintain equipment in working order. In these hospitals, staff members are too rushed to pay attention to frightened patients and lost visitors wandering around in a maze of corridors. Few people smile at strangers or are helpful. In these hospitals, the atmosphere is generally harried and tense. Small wonder, then, that all the marketing budgets in the world don't produce the returns expected.

These organizations have neglected *internal marketing.* They have not created a *customer consciousness.* They have overlooked putting their own house in order before issuing an invitation to outside guests. *Not being customer conscious is a critical failure of many current marketing strategies.*

Before embarking on any marketing strategy, you need to understand that:

- Consumers can only judge the technical and medical competence of a health care facility by the amenities they are directly exposed to. If the TV doesn't work, how do they know that the CAT-scan works properly? If the hospital gets a dinner tray mixed up, how do the consumers know that their lab results won't get mixed up, too?
- Consumers can only judge the competence of a medical facility's staff by the staff that they are in contact with daily and firsthand. If the orderly is gruff or if the nurses are rude and unhelpful, why should the customers believe that their surgeon is competent?
- Consumers today, whether they are buying health care or automobiles, are interested in and demand value for their money. Gone are the days when patients blindly accepted everything that happened to them at the hands of a doctor or hospital. Today, patients question procedures, treatments, and costs. The hospital that can't adequately justify itself will not survive.
- Consumers today are suspicious of advertising that does not deliver the promised results. We live in a post-Ralph Nader world. The hospital that advertises products and services that it can't deliver will lose its customer base to facilities that advertise and do deliver.

The Salesmindedness Imperative

The following situations unfortunately happen far too often in hospitals that have jumped on the marketing bandwagon without careful planning:

- A hospital conducts an advertising campaign that promises free colon cancer screening to anyone who wants it. The calls flood in to the number given. The employees who answer the phone have no idea what the callers are asking for or why the calls are flooding in.
- Newspaper ads announce a brand-new geriatric center at Harkness Hospital. Harkness employees know that no such center exists. The hospital's marketing department has merely bundled several fragmented services together and called it a geriatric center. As a result of the newspaper ad, people call in. Employees have to press the callers for the specific nature of their need so that the employees can direct the callers to the right department of the hospital.
- The new Physician Referral Service has attracted positive public attention. The person staffing it has to take a restroom break. He doesn't bother to forward his phone because he expects to be gone

only a few minutes. The next person to call listens to 15 rings and then hangs up.

- The new cardiac rehabilitation lab opens. The word is out that the fitness equipment is terrific. Employees wonder why they are not allowed to use the equipment.
- One part of the hospital's complex building program is finished at last. Two nursing units are being moved to the new wing today. A visitor arrives at the hospital and asks how to get to her friend's room. The person at the information desk gives her directions to the old wing, which is quite a distance. She arrives at the old wing and finds that her friend isn't there. In fact, the entire nursing unit is empty. She retraces her steps to the information desk. After hearing her dilemma and frustration, the same person who helped her before says, "How was I supposed to know they moved your friend? You never know where people are here from one day to the next."
- The Marketing Department spends a lot of time and money on an elaborate outdoor fair and dedication ceremony to initiate the new physician office building. Few employees attend, and the administration is angry about this apparent lack of support. Rose, a loyal employee, asks, " Were we ever invited?"
- A world-famous doctor has agreed to join the hospital staff. The press hustles to cover this hot story. The next day on the way in to work, Barry from the Maintenance Department is talking with his friend on the bus. His friend says, "Hey, I heard your hospital just got that hotshot surgeon for your staff!" Barry responds, "We did?" and later fumes, "Why does the public know everything before me?" Several days later, the corner butcher tells Barry that he has to have some tests and doesn't know which hospital to go to. Barry replies, "Believe me, if I had a choice of places to go, I wouldn't go there in a million years."

Such stories are all too familiar. These organizations have overlooked the development of *salesmindedness* among their work force. To encourage salesmindedness, which is vital to your hospital's success, remember that:

- New services, strategies, and approaches have to be sold to your employees. If you don't succeed there, you'll have trouble succeeding with your ultimate market: consumers.
- If consumers tell your employees about what's going on in your organization or employees read about what's going on in the newspaper, you'll probably not achieve the customer consciousness you want.

- When employees feel slighted, consumers notice and wonder about your organization.
- When employees are in the dark about a change or service, consumers wonder if your organization knows what it's doing.
- Confused employees confuse your customers. Consumers don't like to be confused, and so they don't want to give you their business.
- Employees implement your plans. Plans don't implement themselves.

Employees deserve to be informed about new services, newsworthy events, procedures for responding to callers, current organizational problems, and more. In fact, they *must* be informed if you expect them to have a stake in supporting and promoting your organization. Without information, employees feel demoralized and discounted.

Informing employees about marketing events and campaigns is important because your employees are megaphones to the outside world. When you communicate well with them, they spread the word about your services and strengths. If you fail to communicate, their misinformation and resentment create obstacles that limit the success of even your most ambitious marketing strategies.

□ All This in a Marketing Framework

By now, marketing is a buzzword in health care. In *The New Hospital* (Rockville, MD: Aspen, 1985), Russell C. Coile, Jr., urges that "for the New Hospital to become a customer-driven organization, it must know who and where its customers are and how to reach them with appropriate marketing strategies. Marketing is not only acceptable but vital. . . . Not all hospitals have willingly embraced marketing, but there will be no escaping it. Those hospitals that first master the new rules of a customer-driven marketplace will definitely have a competitive edge in the future."

So what is *marketing*? Advertising, consumer research, demographics, new product planning, niche building, segmentation, public relations, and sales are all part of the common understanding of marketing and are often used interchangeably. To some organizations, marketing is synonymous with advertising. To others, it's synonymous with sales. To still others, it's the latest word for strategic planning.

For the purposes of this book, *marketing* is a set of organizational practices designed to plan, motivate, and manage the resources and activities of your organization, so that:

- Your organization meets consumer needs and wants.
- The people you want to serve choose your organization for services repeatedly as needed.
- Your organization generates positive opinions of your organization and its services.

Internal Marketing

Internal marketing is a set of practices, processes, and activities designed to develop motivated personnel within an internal environment that builds and supports customer consciousness and sales-mindedness among all personnel. The importance and commitment to internal marketing can be expressed in many ways:

- "The personnel are the first market of the service company." ("Result-Oriented Management by Better Market Orientation or Better Marketing" [English summary], by Christian Groonroos, in the *Finnish Journal of Business Economics*, 4[1981a])
- "Employees precede other publics as the initial market of an organization." ("How to Initiate a Marketing Perspective in a Health Services Organization," by William R. George and Fran Compton, in *Journal of Health Care Marketing*, 1985 Winter, 5[1]:29-37)
- "We can only accomplish our goals through the efforts of our employees. . . . their work, their ideas and commitment." (Quote from R. E. Tallon, executive vice-president at Florida Power and Light, in *Creativity in Services Marketing*, by M. Venkatesan, Diane M. Schmalenser, and Claudia Marshall. Chicago: American Marketing Association, 1986, p. 83)
- "A service firm in order to be successful must first sell the job to its employees in order to sell its services to customers." ("Selling Jobs in the Service Sector," by Earl W. Sasser and Stephen P. Arbeit, in *Business Horizons*, 1987 June, 19[3]:64)
- "Customer-oriented behavior, and thus good interactive marketing performance, cannot be expected unless the firm has something to offer its employees. Internal marketing has to become part of the strategic management philosophy, otherwise more tactical internal marketing activities will be counteracted by demotivating jobs and work environments." ("Internal Marketing: Theory and Practice," by Christian Groonroos, in *Services Marketing in a Changing Environment*, edited by Thomas Block and others. Chicago: American Marketing Association, Proceedings Series, 1985, p. 41)

Internal marketing, then, is a process for establishing, developing,

Chapter 2

and reinforcing excellent customer relations through the organization's own personnel, so that the goals of the customers, the organization, and society are achieved. To effectively conduct internal marketing, the health care organization needs employees and physicians who are *customer oriented* and *salesminded.* Internal marketing is thus a combination of customer consciousness and salesmindedness, as shown in the following formula and in figure 2-1:

> Customer Consciousness + Salesmindedness = Internal
> Marketing Success

Regardless of how you define or look at internal marketing, the bottom line is simple: by satisfying the needs and wants of its internal customers, that is, its employees and physicians, a hospital upgrades its ability to satisfy the needs and wants of its external customers: patients, visitors, third-party payers, and referring physicians.

Figure 2-1. Internal Marketing Process

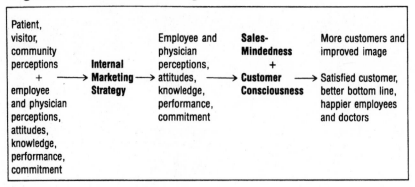

Internal marketing boils down to five truths:

- Personnel are the first market of your organization. If you can't get your employees on your side by behaving with heightened customer consciousness, you will have far-reaching problems satisfying your other customers.
- Employees must understand why they are expected to perform in a certain manner and why you need their support inside and outside the organization.
- You must convince employees of the value of your services if you expect them to support these services in their contacts with customers or prospective customers. According to Frank J. Weaver,

director of public affairs and corporate development for the Cleveland Clinic Foundation in Ohio, 11 percent of consumers select hospitals based on employee recommendations. People believe employees have the inside scoop.

- Employees deliver your services. They need to fully grasp these services and your expectations of them or your intended services never reach the consumer.
- Your information channels must work internally so that your employees can sell externally. Personal selling *to* employees is prerequisite to personal selling *by* employees.

Internal marketing should accomplish the following objectives:

- To help employees understand and accept the importance of their interactions with customers and their responsibility for the total quality, performance, and image of the organization
- To help employees understand and accept the mission, strategies, services, and external campaigns of the organization
- To continuously motivate and train personnel to extend to the organization's diverse customers the communication, compassion, respect, courtesy, and attention they deserve and expect
- To attract and keep excellent employees
- To attract and keep loyal customers

The Tools of Internal Marketing

In "Internal Marketing: Theory and Practice" (in *Services Marketing in a Changing Environment*, edited by Thomas Block and others. Chicago: American Marketing Association, Proceedings Series, 1985), Christian Groonroos outlines several categories of internal marketing activities that his research has indicated are keys to making internal marketing a successful reality. Key activities include the following:

- *Internal training.* Internal training involves training not only personnel who have direct contact with patients and visitors, but also managers and supervisors so that internal marketing is understood and accepted as a function that involves everyone. Employees and physicians also need training in sales techniques and methods for increasing customer satisfaction.
- *Internal face-to-face communication.* Training isn't enough. Managers and supervisors need to continuously interact with their subordinates about service concepts. They need to coach, train, give feedback, and reiterate the importance of customer-oriented

service. Also, they need to establish a climate of open information and communication.

- *Internal mass communication.* Internal mass communication involves internal campaigns that use printed materials, slide shows, and other media to inform employees about service-oriented strategies, promote acceptance, and support managers' efforts to heighten skills.
- *Personnel administration tools.* Personnel tools include hiring practices, job descriptions, wage and salary practices, and the like that are needed to attract and support customer-conscious and salesminded employees.
- *External mass communication and advertising.* At the very least, external advertising campaigns, including brochures and ads, should be presented to employees before they are used externally. Better yet, employees should be involved in their development.
- *Market research.* Market research should be used internally and externally to find out what customers and employees think about the organization's performance in the marketplace.

In "Adapting a Service-Oriented Marketing Strategy in a Service Industry" (in *Service Marketing: Nordic School Perspectives*, edited by Christian Groonroos. Helsingfors, Finland: Swedish School of Economics, 1984, p. 9), C. Ramm-Schmidt asserts that these activities should be integrated into a three-stage process that:

- Analyzes the nature of the service business, including attitudes among employees and customers
- Gets employees to understand how they can become expert at being customer oriented and at internal marketing
- Achieves continuous customer-oriented operations and a perception that high-quality services are being provided

The Chicken or the Egg?

Which comes first, internal or external marketing? The answer is logical. Internal marketing needs to come first. Before you can make an appreciable difference in your bottom line through external marketing campaigns, you need to install a strong, ongoing internal marketing strategy.

If you think that all you need to do is budget for expensive brochures, billboards, full-page ads, and TV commercials, you are making an expensive mistake. Your external marketing efforts will not be successful unless you have marketed to your internal consumers. If patients and other customers coming into the hospital are faced with unfriendly, indifferent, or uninformed staff, they will be tempted to leave or go elsewhere next time no matter how much fancy state-of-the-art equipment you offer. Once again, *internal marketing is not a supplement to external marketing. It is not concurrent with external marketing. It is a prerequisite to external success.*

Keep the following constantly in mind:

• External marketing makes promises.
• Internal marketing keeps promises.

You must be sure you can keep your promises before you risk your credibility making them.

Without internal marketing, the *marketing flow pattern* (figure 2-2) takes over. When you add the internal marketing ingredient, you have revised the marketing flow pattern as shown in figure 2-3. In the revised model, you have added the vital ingredient of alert, skillful, and informed personnel who are rededicated to putting the customer first and are committed to the organization's philosophy and to the value of service excellence.

Figure 2-2. Marketing Flow Pattern

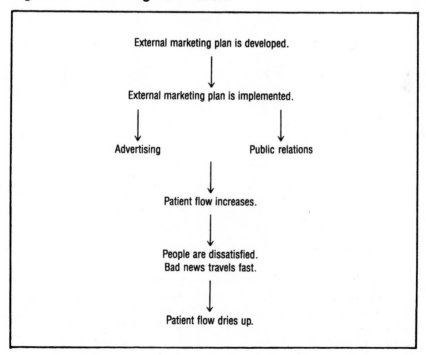

Figure 2-3. Revised Marketing Flow Pattern

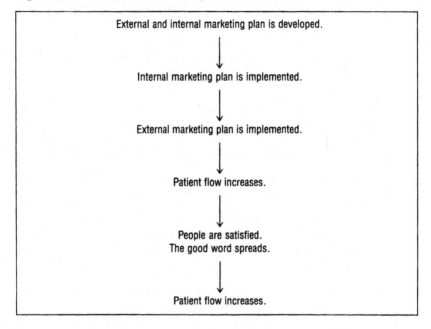

External and internal marketing plan is developed.

↓

Internal marketing plan is implemented.

↓

External marketing plan is implemented.

↓

Patient flow increases.

↓

People are satisfied.
The good word spreads.

↓

Patient flow increases.

☐ The Big Picture

Service organizations, and especially health care organizations, need to include in their marketing activities not only traditional marketing but also internal marketing. Traditional marketing uses the techniques of advertising, selling, promotion, and pricing to determine the organization's marketing mix and to make promises to its prospective customers, who develop expectations based on these promises.

Internal marketing determines the quality of the customer's actual experience with the organization. Customers perceive the organization as a high-quality provider if their experiences match or exceed their expectations. If their experiences are positive, they become an advocate of the organization; happy customers bolster the organization's image and, consequently, affect profitability. However, if they have a negative experience, they may pass on their feelings to other potential customers. This "bad press" may start the organization on a downhill slide that could have serious economic repercussions.

The key to internal marketing in organizations is the emphasis on service excellence. Focusing on service excellence enables health care organizations to meet, and perhaps even surpass, customers' expectations.

A Systems Approach to Service Excellence

☐ Who's the "Customer"?

Considerable debate has occurred on what to call, for lack of a better term, the "health care users." The old incumbent, *patient*, is no longer universally used because it implies that the user is dependent on the health care institution. Many people balk at this implied dependency relationship, especially now that patients are becoming more assertive and active in their own care. Also, if a dependency relationship exists now, it is at least a mutual one. As patients need hospitals, so hospitals need patients to survive. That fact is quite clear.

Although some people still advocate the use of the word *patient*, many people think that an exclusive emphasis on patients in an organization's strategy toward service excellence is too limiting. What about the other customers or users of the organization, such as doctors, family members, visitors, third-party payers, and employees? All of these various constituencies are critical to the organization's success and come to the organization expecting and deserving humane treatment, sensitive service, and attention.

An alternative word is *customer*. After all, users come to hospitals and pay money for services rendered, as in any other business. However, health care isn't like any other business. The term *customer* acknowledges the priority of the user but suggests to many health care workers primarily an economic relationship that may fail to encompass the real, human business of caring, compassion, and healing. The term *customer* may seem to some persons in health care as cold and inappropriate to the special mission that they are there to accomplish. One person launching a strategy to improve service relationships in her hospital crystallized her concern with these words, "I'm sensitive about using the word *customer* because it fuels what is already a top management obsession with the bottom line. Our management forgets that patients are sick people who deserve gentle handling and that employees are by and large hardworking, dedicated individuals motivated to help others. When our management talks only about our 'customers,' they sound as if they are running an organization that produces toaster ovens. I lose confidence in them and feel cynical."

Other words, like *guest, consumer,* and *client* have their pros and cons. In Einstein's national newsletter (*GRIP: Guest Relations in Practice*, 1986 Feb., 1(1):2), readers were asked which term they prefer to use in referring to their users. Of course, rather than resolving the patient-customer-user-consumer-guest-client-patient controversy, the letters received tended only to complicate it. Here are a few examples:

- "We have continued to call our users *patients*, even though the term *client* has been suggested. *Client* has the connotation of a legal or business relationship. *Customer* implies a business or purchasing relationship. Although the term *patient* may seem old-fashioned, I believe it still stands for that special relationship between users and providers of health care. Perhaps we should ask our users which term they prefer." (Helen DeSautel, R.N., M.S., director of patient relations, Baptist Hospital of Miami, Miami, Florida)
- "My suggestion for a term to designate how we regard our patients, guests, or customers is *guest-omer*, a customer who is also our guest. This term recognizes the needs of both. We treat guests in our home differently than we would treat customers at our business. *Guest-omer* recognizes the more intimate relationship we have with our customers in a hospital setting." (Deborah McMann, assistant director, patient relations, University Hospital of Jacksonville, Jacksonville, Florida)
- "The most accurate and realistic term to apply to hospital users should be *victims*. Most consumers of health and medical services have no real choice as to whether—only which. Obviously, preventive services are excluded, but then such services are more concept than reality. Unfortunately." (Richard Gamel, president, MD Search, Inc., Memphis, Tennessee)
- "The discussion concerning the appropriate nomenclature for the

"new" patient/client/customer is so relevant to the issue that I too have spent creative think-time trying to come up with an alternate title. It reminds me of the still unresolved boy/girlfriend/live-in/roommate/housemate/possilq debate. Perhaps we need to consult an anthropologist or a linguist." (Sylvia Wessel)

In the face of continuing controversy, *guest* and *guest relations* have become the terms most frequently used, perhaps because they seem to offer the best compromise. *Guest* is not as harsh a term as *customer* or *user*, and it is more inclusive than *patient* or *client*. Also, it carries the hint of a suggestion that the job of health care organizations is to serve people and satisfy their needs.

However, this book uses the word *customer* because it includes every person with a relationship to the health care organization, including patients, family members, the patient's other visitors and companions, physicians, employees, third-party payers, vendors, and the like. All health care professionals should begin to use the word *customer* without flinching because it is really the clearest and most all-encompassing term. After all, to stay afloat, any organization needs to cater to its customers and satisfy them to the degree humanly and humanely possible. Caring, warmth, and understanding, not just economic power, are intrinsic in its meaning.

Don't let the use of the term *customer*, or even *guest*, fool you. Neither term should imply that hospitals are like hotels. That analogy carried to an extreme is dangerous because hotels and hospitals are really quite different (figure 3-1).

However, the hotel analogy does apply when you think of the guest services that are similar in hotels to hospitals: housekeeping, dietary,

Figure 3-1. Differences between Customers in Hotels and Hospitals

In Hotels	In Hospitals
Most people are there voluntarily.	Health considerations force admission.
Most people are in a good mood.	Most patients feel irritable, exposed, anxious, and scared.
Many people are on expense accounts.	Many patients are panicked about the high cost.
Guests expect pampering and convenience.	Customers expect complex technological know-how to save life and also expect compassion.
Employees must be courteous and responsive.	Employees must be safe, accurate, skilled, careful, compassionate, kind, alert, quick, responsive, and much more.

traffic flow, transportation, maintenance people, amenities, reservations processes, cashiers, checkout, and so forth. But the simple mission of a hotel is service and hospitality. The mission of a hospital is infinitely more complex. Although it does provide service and hospitality, its major concerns include healing, crisis intervention, humanistic dying, and life support. While reading the term *customer* in this book, you must think about it in the fullest sense of the word as it applies to health care.

☐ Understand Who Your Customers Are

Strategically, customers need to be understood as distinct groups with different needs and expectations in relation to health care. For the purposes of this book, consider five key customer segments as the target of strategy for service excellence:

- Patients
- Visitors, family, friends
- Physicians
- The organization's own employees
- Third-party payers

Referral sources and community groups, vendors, volunteers, trustees, and others may also be considered key customer groups by your organization. You need to identify which customer groups to target in your efforts toward service excellence.

Starting with the Obvious—the Patients

Obviously, the first and foremost customer group that is the key to the success of your organization is patients, because they have the most direct and intense experience with your staff and services. For four main reasons, you need to concern yourself with patients' perceptions and patients' satisfaction with your services:

- *The humanistic reason.* Patients deserve excellent quality of care and service because, more often than not, they are quite vulnerable. They come to the hospital when they are sick, worried, pained, concerned, and anxious about their physical, emotional, and economic well-being: "Am I well? Can I get through this emotionally? Can I afford this?" Excellent service is therapeutic.
- *The economic reason.* Patients are customers. They think like customers; they have options that they consider more carefully

than ever; and they expect value for their money.
- *The marketing reason.* Patients are a public relations and sales force. They attract other people to your facility or away from it. They control the grapevine that influences future business.
- *The efficiency reason.* Satisfied patients are easier to serve. Dissatisfied patients consume valuable staff time, time that could be better spent serving more people more thoroughly.

Their Visitors, Family, and Friends

The patient's visitors, family members, and friends are the second key customer group. When they accompany patients to your organization or visit them during their stay, they are frequently overlooked by staff whose primary concern is more often with the patient.

Yet the patient's family and friends also have firsthand experiences with your facility and people. They want their presence and importance to be acknowledged. They want information, and they appreciate comforts, amenities, and updates that help what can be agonizing waits pass more quickly. They may feel edgy, because they feel powerless to help their loved one. Concerned and anxious, they look for information and reassurance themselves. They also act on their protective instincts, by scrutinizing people's behavior toward the patient and by zealously advocating patient's rights.

If family and friends are impressed with their own and their loved one's experience with your organization, they may consider using your facility themselves if they need similar services. However, whether impressed or not, they vociferously spread the word about your organization to the rest of the community. This kind of free advertising can help or hurt your hospital.

The Doctors

Physicians wear two hats: they are care giver and customer. In their customer hat, they have options. If they are not satisfied with the services your organization provides, they can choose the facility down the street. In their care-giver hat, they are also customers in that they rely on your organization's personnel and services to serve their patients.

If you ask physicians about what matters most to them in their relationships with hospitals, they will consistently mention *ease-of-practice* issues. The physician who finds it easy to practice in your organization chooses your organization. An astute strategy for service excellence can help keep doctors satisfied by facilitating the ease with which they practice in the hospital.

Employees

Your own employees also wear two hats: service giver and potential or actual customer. In their role as customer, employees may in fact use your organization for health care when they and their loved ones need it. They also spread the word about your organization to community members, family, and friends; and they field questions about the organization from community members who look to your staff for the inside scoop. To that end, you need to sell your employees on your organization.

Your employees are also service givers who not only provide services to patients, but also provide services to other employees. Employees are internal customers of one another because they rely on one another to get their jobs done. Consequently, a service orientation toward fellow employees is essential. A strategy for service excellence must consider the needs of this important customer group so that they have the stamina and motivation to do their jobs in an excellent manner.

Frank Weaver of the Cleveland Clinic Foundation in Ohio determined that in 1986, 11 percent of hospital users based their choice of a hospital on employee recommendations (figure 1-1). What do your employees say about your organization on the bus ride home, at family gatherings, at community meetings? A trusted information source about your organization, employees deserve to be on the receiving end of services, benefits, information, respect, and care that will inspire productive work on your organization's behalf as well as loyalty and support.

Third-Party Payers

American businesses have figured that health care is an expensive item in their annual budgets. A portion of the price consumers pay for automobiles, airline tickets, and food from fast-food chains, for example, goes to pay for employee health care benefits.

Third-party payers, including businesses, insurance companies, the government, unions, and other health care funders, are shopping for the best health care deals they can find for their constituencies. As they look for the best cost-quality combination, they are looking at individual health care institutions for managed care plans and special deals and services that benefit their employees. They expect service; they expect cost information, answers to their questions, and positive reports from their members about the quality of care and caring received. Your organization has to satisfy these powerful new forces in the health care industry by being responsive to their needs.

□ The Customer Service Matrix

Usually, when people talk about customer relations, they're talking about the interpersonal skills of the health care employee, skills that demonstrate courtesy, compassion, attentiveness, and concern. However, service excellence is more that just people skills. Although your organization's strategy may *start* with a focus on developing employees' interpersonal skills toward patients, your strategy runs the risk of an eventual breakdown and failure unless it addresses service excellence in a much larger context. Strategic approaches to service excellence need to advance an organizationwide commitment to service. When they do, the total service organization is the winner.

The *customer service matrix*, developed by Gail Scott of the Einstein Consulting Group, conveys how comprehensive this service concept needs to be (figure 3-2). Based on an analysis of research identifying the criteria consumers use to evaluate their health care experiences, the customer service matrix defines five key components (vertical axis) integral to service excellence as perceived by each of an organization's key customer groups (horizontal axis).

Figure 3-2.   Customer Service Matrix

Key Components	Customer Groups				
	Patients	Visitors	Physicians	Employees	Third-Party Payers
Technical competence					
Environment					
People skills					
Systems					
Amenities					

An effective strategy for service excellence reflects a lasting commitment to excellent performance on all five components of the customer service matrix:

- *Technical competence.* Technical competence has, more often than not, received the primary focus. Organizations have always been concerned about whether a diagnosis is right, whether laboratory tests are accurate, whether the maintenance worker can fix the air conditioner, and so forth. Increasingly, however, the marketing-oriented health care manager knows that technical competence is not enough, especially because consumers can evaluate this component less well than they can evaluate other, more familiar aspects of service, like friendliness, respectful treatment, easy access, attentiveness, and convenience.

- *People skills.* The surge of interest in customer relations has focused primarily on people skills, specifically the courtesy, care, and concern that personnel in the organization extend to patients, visitors, physicians, and one another. No doubt, people skills have a dramatic impact on consumer satisfaction, the reputation of the organization that spreads through the grapevine, and the consumer's future choices about where to go for care. A rude receptionist can turn away a patient faster than parking problems and even a fuzzy diagnosis.
- *Environment.* The physical environment also merits attention. Many who have instituted customer relations programs have unearthed parking, transport, and physical access problems that frustrate customers and turn them away. Employees feel that more courteous behavior on their part does not adequately compensate for environmental problems, nor should they have to bend over backward to compensate for management's neglect of these factors. Organizations with dilapidated, dirty, or unsafe buildings dissuade patients from returning. How comfortable can a patient and visitor feel and how energetic do physicians and employees feel in an unappetizing environment? The physical environment, its accessibility and aesthetics, deserves consideration as part of a comprehensive strategy for service excellence.
- *Systems.* Even people skills are not enough unless underlying systems support them. Many customer relations programs come to a crashing halt because of inattention to this component. Employees get frustrated apologizing to patients for long waits day after day and year after year. Especially in an atmosphere of increased concern for the customer, these employees resent underlying systems problems and inconveniences that interfere with their ability to extend the care and attention they want to extend to customers. Long waits, cumbersome and interminable decision-making processes, equipment that doesn't work, poor scheduling practices, circuitous routes from one location to another, and the perennial absence of supplies when you need them are all examples of lapses in support systems.

Without attention to underlying systems problems, good employees gradually become demoralized and less effective in people skills. Also, the organization's relationships with employees are perceived as poor by the customer, who has been oppressed by the organization's senseless procedures and practices and drained of time, energy, and patience.

- *Amenities.* Amenities that an organization can provide its customers, such as coffee in the waiting room, trinkets and a play area for the kids, a Walkman® in the dental chair, free toothbrush and shampoo in an attractive container, valet parking, videocassette recorders, and colorful linens, make customers feel more comfortable and special. However, although such amenities may be appreciated by customers, they do not compensate for other service deficiencies. Patients complain bitterly that although the pile of magazines in the waiting room may make the time go faster, they should still not have to suffer long waits (caused by a systems problem) or rude employees (caused by poor people skills). Attention to amenities to the exclusion of a hard-nosed attack on systems problems, such as long waits or misplaced charts and laboratory tests, is misguided and limits the long-term success of your organization's strategy for service excellence.

Health care leaders need to make conscious decisions on how their organization rates on each service component in relation to each key customer group. To plan a comprehensive, long-term, strategy for service excellence, follow these three key steps:

- Identify your key customer groups and their needs and expectations.
- Evaluate your organization along the five major components of service excellence for each key customer group. Solicit information from each customer group about their likes and dislikes to help you set priorities.
- Generate a phased, long-term strategy for building on strengths and overcoming weaknesses.

□ Systems Approach a Must

> For every complex problem, there's a simple solution, and it's wrong.
>
> —H. L. Mencken

An organizationwide effort or *systems approach* is needed if your organization is to reap long-term, tangible results. Many forces in the organization—such as personnel policies and practices, top management philosophy and practices, messages on the walls, behavior of department heads and supervisors, nature of job expectations, hiring practices, communication systems, and scope and frequency of training and skill building—directly influence employee behavior and consequently indirectly affect customer perceptions of employee behavior. All of these influencing forces have to push in the same direction. If they don't, if they push for conflicting behavior or communicate double messages, employees are thrown into an impossible bind. They get angry and rightfully so.

At Einstein, we learned this the hard way. When we were first trying to figure out how to improve customer relations at our hospital, we started by developing a nitty-gritty skill-building program for admissions representatives. We decided that we should start where patients start, at the front door, and help employees who have first contact with patients demonstrate excellent skills that get the patient experience off to a good start. We developed a compact and engaging training program to help admissions representatives meet and greet, make small talk with nervous people, take the initiative to make people comfortable, anticipate needs, and ease a patient's long wait. We thought that concrete, relevant skills could be taught, and so did the admissions representatives. The program was successful. Admissions representatives appreciated such job-specific skill building, and they felt important because of the revived focus on customer relations.

Two weeks later, Martha, an admissions representative, called me and said, "Remember that great program you ran for us?" Proudly, I said, "Sure!" She went on to explain that her supervisor had disciplined her because of it. Because Martha was freshly aware of customer relations, she actively seized opportunities to make patients comfortable. One day, she noticed an anxious older woman who waited alone to be admitted. The woman was shaking and teary-eyed. Martha left her cubicle and sat down with the woman, put her hand on her arm, talked with her, and tried to ease her aloneness and her admitted fright about her hospital stay.

Martha's supervisor didn't like what Martha had done. She called Martha into her office and said, "What do you think you're doing making chit-chat with that little old lady when we have people to admit. Don't you know you're supposed to see six people an hour, ten minutes per person?"

So Martha was caught between pressure from her supervisor to be productive at all costs, and pressure from me and our customer relations training agenda to cater to distressed patients at all costs. As you can imagine, Martha was distraught because she thought she had done the right thing.

This upsetting sequence of events led us to an invaluable and far-reaching realization. Training is only a Band-Aid® unless the system supports and reinforces the employees' new behavior. Martha was a training success story until she tried to do what she had learned, did it well, and was punished for it. When that happened, we realized that we had to slow down on the training and take a look at all hospital systems that shape behavior.

The employee shouldn't be the victim of a conflict between the supervisor's objectives and the objectives of customer relations training. Top management has to decide what they really want from employees and then get their middle managers and line supervisors to support this objective and make it happen. Perhaps management can encourage personnel to put a dual value on productivity and customer relations, or perhaps productivity should be secondary when a particular patient is suffering. The point is that the powers-that-be have to decide what they want; they must decide which priorities should be driving both the system and employee behavior. Then training can be developed to support those values and help people achieve service excellence.

Think of the hospital as a temple dedicated to customer satisfaction and high-quality care. The forces in the system that shape employee behavior are the pillars that support the temple. If the pillars are not in place, the temple falls. Ten pillars in particular are essential to support service excellence. These pillars are introduced in chapter 4 and examined in depth in part II of this book.

Without a systems approach that deliberately builds these pillars of support, you run the great risk of creating impossible internal conflicts in your organization, conflicts that place employees in unmanageable binds and generate intolerable frustration. The result is that people will be jumping off the service excellence bandwagon just as you're trying to drive it forward.

To promote a systems approach, ask yourself:

- What forces in this organization influence employee behavior?
- Which forces are already working for excellent service, and how can you capitalize on these?
- Which forces are working against excellent service?
- How can you realign these forces so that they no longer push against service excellence but instead support it?

□ An Ongoing Process

The achievement of service excellence is a process, not a program. A program has a beginning and an end, like a political campaign. If service excellence were simply a program, you could find yourself a glitzy name and circulate nice posters and distribute buttons. You could push it vehemently for a year, and then you could move on.

However, service excellence should not be considered a program. It is not a discrete event but a strategic way of doing business. It should be a *value* in the culture of the hospital. It needs to be firmly installed and actively and aggressively maintained *forever*. After building a customer-consciousness mind set among your people, you have to enforce and reinforce it over the long haul.

Consider quality of care. Would you ever say, "We had a quality of care program last year, and now we're moving on to something else?" The same is true of service excellence. It needs to be a value that drives people and the system, and it needs to be nurtured and fed or it fades.

Service excellence involves continual efforts to understand the degree of satisfaction felt by each key customer group, to evaluate trade-offs and possible improvements (their costs and benefits), and to commit resources to incremental improvements and refinements as needs and perceptions change. For example, Harper Hospital (a fictitious name) gave extensive 16-hour customer relations training to its 2,200 employees. Although behavior reportedly changed temporarily, systems problems that had been neglected demoralized the newly trained employees. With their heightened consumer consciousness, they, like consumers, had no further tolerance for systems problems that oppressed people. In fact, the employees were angry that skill training had been provided without devoting one iota of effort to what they perceived to be causal problems. Employees felt that management blamed patient dissatisfaction on poor employee skills, when employees saw the barriers to customer satisfaction quite differently. In this case, a staff skill-building strategy was instituted before the crux of the hospital's service problems were pinpointed. Not surprisingly, the proposed solution—a training program—failed to make the intended changes happen.

If you take the time to analyze the big picture, you lower the risk of making false starts or insignificant moves in your efforts to achieve service excellence. You avoid the risk of trying out easy, but myopic, improvements.

Sometimes, a value takes a long time to become part of an organization. However, the longer it takes, the more solid the change. Some hospitals create an all-out, dynamic campaign for customer relations. An enthusiastic, energetic committee does all it can as fast as it can but then runs out of steam and strategies. Awareness dims, and people get frustrated. They moved too fast. Service excellence is not a now-or-never process; it is a *long-term forever process.*

No Less than a Culture Change

Health care organizations used to be able to set the rules and expect consumers to conform to them. Reimbursement was nearly infinite and automatic, and there were plenty of patients to go around. In many organizations that started as charity institutions, employees subtly conveyed the attitude that consumers should be grateful to them. For example, hospitals had no weekend hours for outpatient services because staff found weekend hours inconvenient. The provider's preferences ruled, and the consumer went along. But times have changed.

Provider-oriented cultures are changing into consumer-oriented cultures if an organization wants to move ahead. Such culture changes require new values, new rhetoric, and a revamping of "the way things are done around here."

What's involved in culture change? Plenty. Years ago, behavioral scientist Kurt Lewin described organizational change as a three-step sequential process, and this process describes culture change as well:

- *Unfreezing:* thawing out established behavior patterns
- *Changing:* moving to a new pattern
- *Refreezing:* maintaining the new pattern

Unfreezing (step 1) is typically and inevitably unsettling and stems from tensions that drive people to search for new approaches. Such tension often develops from a financial downturn, image problems, falling standards, competitive pressures, and the like. If your people don't feel this tension, you have to take explicit steps to create mild states of anxiety, or your people won't be motivated to change. That's why service improvement strategies should not shelter employees from the anxiety-provoking facts of today's environment. Edgar Schein puts it this way: "One simply cannot change pieces of a stable culture without creating potential mass anxiety" ("What You Need to Know about Organizational Culture,' *Training and Development Journal*, 1986 Jan., 40[1]:30-33). Schein goes on to say that "unfreezing includes the pain of disconfirmation—old assumptions no longer work. Leadership is critical at this stage; it is required to help the group cope with and not avoid anxiety. Leaders not only develop and articulate new visions but they create trust. They help members of the group to survive the anxieties that accompany transitions."

An effective strategy for service excellence cannot be simply a morale-boosting, foot-stomping barrel of fun. If it is, you run the risk of installing a superficial program that does not trigger the reexamination and redirection of the culture necessary to make substantive change happen.

The Stretch from Good to Excellent

How far must people really stretch to provide service excellence? This question is a difficult one. Figure 3-3 attempts an answer.

Figure 3-3. Is Excellence Possible?

From the Editor

Dear Readers,

I overheard a vehement argument the other day. The question boiled down to this: Is excellence possible in today's health care environment?

Frankly, while I felt quite opinionated about the subject at the outset, I ended up in a quandary, feeling as the debate fizzled that the jury is still out on this one! Here's the gist of it. To protect the innocent, I'll call the two parties involved "YAY" and "NAY" based on their overall responses to the question.

YAY: Excellence is certainly possible! It's a relative thing that always exists within parameters or constraints. With DRGs, cutbacks, changing hospital usage patterns, and other new facts of hospital life, the parameters and constraints have changed. Within these new boundaries, excellence is still possible. It just looks different than it may have looked in the past.

NAY: That's an unbelievable rationalization. You're just weakening your definition of excellence so you can still say excellence is possible. Excellence is not a relative thing. Excellence is the best we can imagine doing. Let's get down to basics and stop the semantic games! Start with a patient, a very sick, very scared patient, a patient who's also alone. You have a nurse rushing around with more patients than ever and sicker patients than ever. That nurse has limited time and can't, no matter how much she or he *wants* to do for that patient, do everything that patient needs. How can you possibly say excellence is happening in that case?

YAY: Time is a quality issue, not a quantity issue. It's the same in parenting. You can have a parent who's with a child all day and that parent is mildly distracted, not really attending to the child, easily irritated, and quick to pounce on the child's every utterance. Then you have the parent who spends 30 great minutes a day, focusing on the child, listening, really tuning in. I am convinced that parent number two is excellent and parent number one is not.

NAY: But what if parent number two's child has special needs that don't precisely fit into the 30 minutes that parent has decided to devote to the child? Same in hospitals. The patient has needs, and that nurse must have the flexibility to respond to those needs in ways that might not exactly fit into the nurse's tight time constraints. So the backrub that could do wonders for a patient just doesn't happen. The fact that it can't happen moves that nurse down the excellence continuum, even though that nurse can't be blamed for it.

YAY: I'll admit here that there may not be time for that backrub, no matter how efficient

(continued)

Figure 3-3. *(continued)*

the nurse is. But, once you accept time as an excuse for mediocrity, you're doing what so many health care employees are doing nowadays, using time as a cop-out. Look at guest relations. When a hospital is installing higher standards of guest relations, a typical form of resistance is "we don't have time." Thinking the way you do, you would probably accept this excuse and be too timid to set high standards of behavior toward hospital guests.

NAY: No, I wouldn't. I'd say that within the time constraints, you can and should extend yourself to patients with superior courtesy, compassion, respect, and attentiveness.

YAY: Right! You're agreeing with me, then, that excellence is something that can happen within whatever constraints you have to accept. I say, first push the constraints and do all you can to expand them, using creativity and innovative ways to do what you know you need to do for the patient's sake. Once you've stretched the constraints so that you have maximum room to meet patient needs, then excellence is defined within those bounds.

NAY: I still think you're selling out. Don't you think there is an objectively excellent way to care for a person and your "bounds" may make that way of caring out of the question?

YAY: Maybe so, but why beat ourselves over the head with what we can't do? Why not make the most of what we can?

NAY: I agree with you there. But don't call that excellence.

YAY: Look at it a different way for a minute. Do you admit that DRGs have caused hospitals to change internal systems and procedures?

NAY: Sure. So what?

YAY: We've had to reexamine old practices and make some changes that increase efficiencies, get patients home sooner. And we've had to ask ourselves if everything we do for patients is really in their best interest. I honestly think that, as a result, many positive changes have taken place that are good for patients. I doubt very much that we do as many unnecessary procedures as we used to or that we keep as many people in the alien hospital environment too long. We've been forced to get the slack out of the hospital rope with some very good effects. And as a result, we're approaching excellence.

NAY: You're a very creative rationalizer.

YAY: You might think that. I'm saying that excellence is a goal that motivates positive, ongoing changes. Look at Tom Peters' book. The name is *In Search of Excellence;* it is not *This Is Excellence!* Everybody's searching for it. It's not a clear, tangible, concrete thing. And within the new constraints we now have, we also have new opportunities that drive us toward excellence in new ways.

NAY: Maybe you're right. Maybe not.

Let's put it to the jury. Readers, what do you think? Is excellence possible?

Sincerely,

Wendy Leebov, Editor.

Reprinted with permission from *Guest Relations in Practice* (1987 Jan.-Feb. 2[1]:1-4).

If you don't strive for excellence, whether or not it's possible to achieve, you are doomed to fail in your efforts to motivate your work force. Picture a continuum of employee behavior from awful on the left to great and impressive on the right, with inoffensive, good, and very good in between (figure 3-4). Many management teams are interested in customer relations because they are tired of the small number of people at the left end of the continuum, the customer relations offenders. These people are rude, inattentive, indifferent, or irritable; they cause vehement complaints, guest dissatisfaction, time-consuming troubleshooting, and image problems. If only these people would shape up, thinks management, the organization's image would be so much improved. Managers who want a strategy for service excellence that will rehabilitate or get rid of these people have one goal—to stop offensive, expensive behavior. In fact, many organizations devote resources to customer relations for just this reason. In a culture that has rarely disciplined employees for mediocre or worse interpersonal skills, such a goal is not unusual. However, it is short-sighted.

Figure 3-4. Continuum of Employee Behavior toward Customers

Continuum of Employee Behavior				
Awful	Inoffensive	Good	Very Good	Great

Objectives for service excellence need to be ambitious and inspirational. If you move people successfully from awful to inoffensive or even good, you've come some distance, and the temptation is to feel satisfied because the elimination of offensive behavior also quiets the many complaints you had to handle previously. A facade of positivity exists because of the absence of negativity. However, the absence of negativity does not mean positivity. By reaching for "goodness" and not "excellence," you limit the potential of your strategy for service excellence in two far-reaching ways:

- People are only inspired when they strive toward excellence.
- Striving for inoffensiveness is not inspirational.

Being "good" does not help your organization. In a competitive environment, goodness is not good enough. The competitive edge is *excellence*. Service does not stand out as a competitive strength unless it's so strong in your organization that it captures the attention of the consumer. You have to be great for the consumer to notice, not just okay. You have to exceed the consumers' expectations to the point where they stop short and are impressed by how good you really are.

Too many hospitals don't reach high enough. When initial efforts reduce complaints about offensive behavior, they feel an aura of success. Management relaxes its efforts and commitment because of a reduction of complaints. Your message should be to settle for nothing less than excellence. Your message should be:

> Good isn't good enough for us. This organization is too good to set our sights on being merely decent to people. We want to *stand out* in our treatment of customers. Only through excellence can we give our customers the treatment they deserve. Only through excellence can customer relations bring us customers. Only through excellence can we maintain our own integrity as health care givers and hold in high esteem our workplace and ourselves.

The Foundation for Service Excellence

The Story of Two Carpenters
One carpenter was wise. She took a long time to anchor her house on a solid foundation. The other carpenter was foolish. This carpenter was in a hurry. "Foundations are not important," he thought, "except in a storm and a storm may never come." So, he built his house on insecure footings. The ensuing storm blew the house down.

Picture your carefully architectured strategy for service excellence as a temple constructed to withstand the ravages of time. At the first rumble of pressure, will your temple hold up, or will it start to crumble? One misplay by a member of your service excellence team and tenets that form your finely conceived structure can start to chip away. So how do you keep the structure intact? By developing a strong, long-term support system—the 10 pillars of service excellence.

- Management philosophy and commitment
- Accountability
- Input and evaluation
- Problem-solving and complaint management
- Downward communication
- Staff development and training
- Physician involvement
- Reward and recognition
- Employee as customer
- Reminders, refreshers, attention grabbers

These 10 pillars represent 10 powerful forces, all of which need to be pointed in the same direction. These pillars are the primary forces that determine your degree of success, and so each pillar must be solid, long-lasting, and supportive of your quest for service excellence.

☐ Pillar 1. Management Philosophy and Commitment

The first pillar necessary to support your strategy for service excellence is *management philosophy and commitment.* Service excellence can't survive if it is conceived as only a program. It needs to be an organizational value and a commitment that is pervasive at every level of the organization. Such a commitment takes leadership, and courageous leadership at that. Top management needs to stick its proverbial neck out if people are going to be moved toward service excellence.

Pick up the latest writing of management gurus Tom Peters *(Passion for Excellence),* Richard S. Ruch and Ronald Goodman *(Image at the Top: Crisis and Renaissance in Corporate Leadership),* Terrence E. Deal and Allan A. Kennedy *(Corporate Cultures: The Rites and Rituals of Corporate Life),* and Harvey Hornstein *(Managerial Courage).* They and numerous others all espouse the need for value-driven organizations. Employees, especially health care employees, want to identify with an organization that is striving to exemplify values they believe in. Values motivate and inspire if management communicates those values, exemplifies them, and reinforces them repeatedly in decisions and resource allocations. Strategies for service excellence need to be driven specifically by an explicit value on service excellence.

The power of strong top management commitment is obvious. Moderate commitment can work in some cases if top management is ready with support when it's needed. However, the lack of strong commitment sends your strategy into the danger zone. When departments won't schedule their people into a mandatory workshop, when extra dollars are needed to fund a recognition strategy, when two department heads won't set ambitious service standards with their people because they don't work with patients, when employees have ideas about ways to improve service but no one will listen, that's when your strategy starts to crack and crumble.

Management commitment is not an elusive force. Chapter 5 explores the intricacies of knowing when it's there and building it brick by brick. Specifically, the chapter examines:

- Management language: mission and value statements
- The power of management as role models
- The standard-setting process
- Management visibility and availability
- The manager's role in follow-through
- Search for opportunities for active involvement
- Use of administrative clout to inspire cooperation
- The role of truth telling in service excellence
- Their key role in building support systems for problem solving and communication
- Overall openness and willingness to take risks

Management involvement and commitment is a tall but achievable order for the forward-looking, forward-moving administrator or administrative team.

☐ Pillar 2. Accountability

The second pillar is *accountability.* Personnel practices must be on the same high level as the standards set for your strategy for service excellence. These standards need "teeth"; they need built-in accountability systems that say, for example: if a certain cleanup responsibility is ignored, then James W., the first-floor maintenance worker, will be held accountable.

What are some of your options in addressing the accountability issue? You can write a policy that explicitly builds service expectations into every job in the hospital. Let everyone know what they're expected to do, not just what they're not to do.

You can rewrite each job description and include service requirements that are appropriate for each job. Job descriptions don't have to be the time-worn compilation of technical skills. They can and should include appropriate customer relations behaviors, such as putting the patient's food tray within reach of the patient.

You can examine your performance appraisal system. Does service-oriented behavior receive adequate attention, or are evaluations bogged down with vague words like *attitude* and *human relations* that blur the actual behaviors you want to encourage?

Perhaps the first impression the patient receives when arriving at the hospital is at the admissions desk. The admission officers as well as the long line of hospital personnel that follows (for example, transporters, tray personnel, maintenance people) all have unique opportunities to create positive patient relationships. Middle managers and supervisors should be taught how to communicate customer relations expectations to their subordinates and reinforce them through positive recognition, coaching, and progressive disciplinary measures, when necessary.

Chapter 6 examines eight key ways to build accountability for service excellence in your organization:

- Creating a systemwide policy for service excellence
- Issuing explicit expectations for employee behavior
- Building service expectations into job descriptions
- Building service dimensions into your performance appraisal process
- Hiring the right people in the first place
- Getting new people off on the right foot through your new-employee orientation
- Developing a formal commendation process
- Educating your management and supervisory personnel about how to use the system

☐ Pillar 3. Input and Evaluation

Once you've installed your strategy for service excellence, how can you be sure that you're advancing toward excellent customer relations? Without built-in systems for ongoing *input and evaluation*, the third pillar, you can't be sure how you're doing or what you need to do next. This pillar focuses on your systems for gathering input from your key customer groups and evaluating their degree of satisfaction with your people and services. Your overall service strategy needs to be guided by evaluation data that are readily and consistently available. Otherwise, you're navigating blindly, not to mention missing invaluable opportunities to gain constructive feedback.

Often patient representatives and marketing department people have already installed illuminating input-gathering devices. Chapter 7 discusses multiple ways to tap into each customer group using quite a variety of methods, including focus groups, surveys, interviews, audits, complaint tracking, and the like. Specifically, you'll see options for learning not only from patients, but also from visitors, employees, physicians, and third-party payers.

☐ Pillar 4. Problem Solving and Complaint Management

The fourth pillar refers to *problem solving and complaint manage-*

ment. Timely and organized systems for handling complaints, systems problems, and sorely needed improvements increase customer satisfaction.

What happens in your organization when people complain? Does someone or some group look at the complaint and figure out how to prevent the problem in the future? When people point to service weaknesses or make suggestions about how to make things better, what happens to their input? Systems and procedures that don't work must be weeded out and dealt with promptly before they have an opportunity to threaten your strategy and your employees' morale. Maybe the problem is a faulty scheduling system that subjects the patient to repeated long waits, an inefficient billing procedure, or a broken vending machine in the employee lounge. Whatever the problem, neither customer nor employee should find something in obvious need of change, tell you about it, and then watch their input being ignored.

Imagine a hospital in which all staff members excel in people skills. Everyone's gracious, respectful, and sensitive to the needs of patients, visitors, and colleagues. However, the hospital is plagued by systems problems. People always have to wait because of understaffing or poor scheduling procedures, the emergency room or front lobby never has enough wheelchairs, charts are lost, computers are down, medications aren't delivered at night, orders are mixed up, the quantity of bed linens is never sufficient, people wait endlessly to be assigned a room, and on and on.

When a hospital has systems problems, all of its key customer groups are victims: patients aren't happy, visitors aren't happy, physicians aren't happy, and employees are likely to be downright angry. Your organization needs to pay systematic attention to solving systems problems and to refining systems so that they are accessible, convenient, user friendly, and responsive to customers.

Pillar 3, input and evaluation, involves ways to generate data or input from every one of your key customer groups. But then what happens with those data? Unless you funnel them into problem-solving processes or into the hands of people with the power to listen and act, you are doing nothing more than inviting your customers to vent so that you can appease them.

If you don't have reliable mechanisms for reviewing, problem solving, and acting on input from customers, you lose out on opportunities to improve your organization and tackle the problems that dissatisfy your customers. You also make people, especially employees and physicians, angry. Employers and physicians quickly learn that, although you ask what they think, you do not intend to do anything about it. Instead, their valuable perspectives and ideas are filed in someone's circular file or met with "I'll get back to you." No one ever does, and the problem lives on.

Drawing on the wealth of experience contributed by patient representatives, chapter 8 lays out a variety of mechanisms for effective problem-solving and complaint management, mechanisms that digest, set priorities, and process the riches of customer complaints, perceptions, and preferences. It also takes a hard look at the problems hospitals seem to have in tackling systems problems, the organizational obstacles that make these problems seem insurmountable, and a variety of strategies for making your organization user friendly.

☐ Pillar 5. Systems for Downward Communication

"Nobody ever tells me anything!" Have you ever heard this said by employees or physicians in your organization? The fifth pillar, *downward communication*, attacks this problem.

Employee attitude surveys show that employee morale is defeated more by no news than by bad news. Organizations want employees and doctors to be invested in and committed to their organizations, but why should they if the people at the top don't keep them informed about how the organization is doing, what people are doing, and how they can help. Also, what is happening as a result of their efforts on the organization's behalf and as a result of their complaints, suggestions, and innovative ideas? In an information vacuum, key people feel ignored, unacknowledged, and unvalued.

Chapter 9 examines in greater depth your options for strengthening or building, once and for all, downward communication systems that keep your key people informed. A variety of methods are presented with examples of how these methods have worked in other organizations.

☐ Pillar 6. Staff Development and Training

Service excellence as a separate field of study is still in swaddling clothes. Even people who are disciplined and well motivated, like that seasoned 30-year veteran who's never ruffled any feathers, may need special training and skill building in interpersonal skills to move from "good" to "excellent."

The sixth pillar, *staff development and training*, helps people sharpen their skills in the art of meeting and greeting, extending empathy, handling complaints, easing long waits, making small talk to ease anxiety, and even in just plain listening. A small hug, when the occasion calls for it, speaks volumes.

Your service excellence or customer relations steering committee or coordinator needs to evaluate potential training resources both outside as well as within the organization to decide on a suitable long-term training agenda and to determine the training priorities for each department or layer. Chapter 10 explores in depth a wide variety of needs for awareness raising and skill building and outlines a diverse training agenda that moves your people from "good" to "great" and from "inoffensive" to "noticeably impressive" in customer relations skills. Specifically, you'll find help in kicking off your strategy for service excellence and developing training programs for administrators, department heads and supervisors, nurses, front-line employees, people with substantial telephone responsibility, people who have but a minute with the patient, job-specific groups, and many others in the hospital.

☐ Pillar 7. Physician Involvement

Two hats and a hands-off tradition make *physician involvement*, the seventh pillar, difficult. The physician's number-one hat is as a customer who has what is often a vast choice among hospitals. If your hospital doesn't treat physicians right—for example, with quick turnaround of lab results, easy and quick admission of their patients, cooperative nurses, accommodating medical clerks, support in attracting patients, referrals, a nice lounge, and the like—then the physician may just admit patients to St. Down the Block.

When wearing hat number two, physicians are part of your care team and, like employees, need to demonstrate caring, compassionate, and courteous behavior to hospital guests, and these guests include employees. Also, if physicians are in no way involved in your strategy for service excellence, employees will understandably be resentful and use this resentment as the reason to limit their own cooperation with higher service standards because they see the old double standard rearing its ugly head.

One way or another then, physicians must be part of your strategy for service excellence. As customers, they can help you identify the aspects of your services that attract or repel them and their patients. As care givers, they need to be exposed to the new higher standards of service behavior and to be made aware of the numerous benefits to be gained from conformity, along with all other hospital staff members, to these new standards.

Chapter 11 does exploratory surgery on physician involvement. It examines:

- The nuances of the different groups (attending physicians, residents, and employed physicians)
- The critical role of physician liaison
- Methods for involving them in planning their own involvement
- Optional approaches and interventions
- Effective pitches and appeals

☐ Pillar 8. Reward and Recognition

Excellence in service may be its own reward, but it's better to assume that it isn't. As part of your strategy, you need to bestow *rewards and recognition*, the eighth pillar, on those who deserve it, those who have distinguished themselves by their exemplary energy, behavior, and sense of commitment.

Do you already have a reward and recognition system? Does it reinforce the behavior patterns expected in your strategy for service excellence? Are groups, departments, and individuals all included in the acknowledgment process?

An employee-of-the-month program is fine as far as it goes. However, your objective is to create many winners, not just a select few. Chapter 12 examines a smorgasbord of strategies for recognizing and rewarding employees for small feats, minor miracles, and other demonstrations of service excellence.

☐ Pillar 9. Employee as Customer

Happy employees make patients happy. Conversely, if your employees are demoralized or feel unappreciated and devalued in your environment, they are hardly able or likely to win over patients for your organization. To sustain a satisfied and productive work force, you have to make your workplace a nourishing place to work.

The ninth pillar, *employee as customer*, looks at the key components involved in treating your employees as customers whose needs must be understood and addressed in order to engender employee satisfaction. Chapter 13 provides methods for doing just this and shares examples of campaigns and approaches aimed at the employee as customer.

☐ Pillar 10: Reminders, Refreshers, and Attention Grabbers

Time passes, and awareness fades. A whole host of other problems and pressures clutter people's already overcrowded heads. This situation is what makes the tenth pillar, *reminders, refreshers, and attention grabbers,* so important.

You have to take action to remind people of your service priority and to refresh their minds, mind set, and approaches. You're in competition for people's attention, and so you have to consciously institute methods that trigger attention to service excellence. Otherwise well-intentioned people with their hearts in the right place just may not be thinking about it.

Chapter 14 describes a rich variety of ways to pull people's attention to service excellence periodically so that service excellence is not a stale or disappearing theme. You'll find ideas about visual reminders, such as posters, buttons, T-shirts, and the like, and energizers, such as contests, special events, refresher programs, organizationwide workshops, or rituals that revive awareness and commitment.

☐ Strong Pillars Make for Strong Institutions

The next 10 chapters of this book explore the 10 pillars one by one. You will find a rationale for each pillar as well as alternative approaches, illustrations, and suggestions.

Note, please, that these pillars are not sequential or chronological. You may choose to read them according to your interests or in any order that appeals to you.

If your customer relations strategy or strategy for service excellence is already in place, you should read with an eye toward identifying gaps or the telltale signs of crumbling pillars. If you have no strategy in place yet, let these pillars catapult you forward in planning a comprehensive, well-supported strategy.

With your 10 pillars firmly grounded, your "temple" to service excellence will be an enduring credit to all those who have contributed to its successful design, construction, and maintenance.

□Part Two

The 10 Pillars of Service Excellence

□ **Chapter 5**

Management Philosophy and Commitment

For an enlightening experiment, take the self-test in figure 5-1 before you read this chapter. Make 16 copies of this inventory, and ask a variety of people including 3 administrators, 5 department heads, and 8 nonsupervisory employees to fill it out from their perspectives. Then count the number of "yes" answers. If the average score is below 12, you need to do some serious work at the management level if you want to bolster your strategy for service excellence. If your score is anything less than perfect, look at your "no" answers, and you'll know what you have to do.

The results of this test should give you a clear picture of the degree to which management philosophy and practices support service excellence. These results and the information in this chapter can help you engage your management team in a reexamination of the strategic importance they assign to service excellence in your organization.

□ Management's Role in Service Excellence

A license examiner was giving a test to new drivers. Among the questions was this one: "What is the most dangerous part of the car?" The child in the backseat piped up, "The driver."

Just as the child said, the "driver," or in this case the management team, is the most dangerous and most important element because if

Figure 5-1.   Self-Test: How Solid Is Management Support?

Management Philosophy and Commitment. Circle the appropriate answer. The more "yes" answers, the better. "No" answers indicate areas that need improvement.

1. Administrators frequently refer to service excellence and patient satisfaction as driving forces in your organization's culture.   Yes   No

2. Managers and supervisors who are technically competent, but negative in their interpersonal skills toward employees, patients, and doctors, are under pressure from the top to meet standards for service excellence.   Yes   No

3. Generally, top administrators show courtesy, friendliness, and a caring attitude toward patients and visitors.   Yes   No

4. Generally, top administrators show courtesy, friendliness, and a caring attitude toward employees.   Yes   No

5. Managers and supervisors are helped by their bosses to be role models of customer relations excellence.   Yes   No

6. Administrators have communicated clear expectations to department heads regarding the middle manager's role in strengthening service standards and practices.   Yes   No

7. Administrators, department heads, and supervisors are encouraged to coach, discipline and, if needed, terminate employees who persist in their failure to meet high standards for service excellence.   Yes   No

8. Administrators, department heads, and supervisors have established and communicated clear, job-specific expectations to the people they supervise.   Yes   No

9. Administrators, middle managers, and supervisors hold employees accountable for their behavior toward customers and confront problem employees when such employees tarnish the organization's image.   Yes   No

10. The in-house customer relations coordinator gets support and cooperation from management.   Yes   No

11. Administrators here view service excellence as an organizationwide priority, not just the job of a particular person or department.   Yes   No

(continued)

Figure 5-1. *(continued)*

12. The organization's budget reflects a commitment to
    service excellence and customer relations.   Yes   No

13. Management has established systems for employee
    input.   Yes   No

14. Management has established ongoing processes for
    tackling problems that frustrate employees.   Yes   No

15. Administrators communicate downward on a
    regular basis.   Yes   No

16. Administrators show respect toward employees by
    sharing information about the organization's
    mission, philosophy, progress, and problems.   Yes   No

                                          Total: ___   ___

you don't have top-management support, you don't have a strategy for service excellence. Obviously, management support involves more than signing memos, attending workshops, and allocating money. Ideally, starting with the top executives, managers need to *lead* your strategy for service excellence and behave as organizational champions for this espoused value.

Consider the wisdom of management gurus Tom Peters *(In Search of Excellence)* and Clay Sherman *(The Uncommon Leader)*. Peters asserts the need for "organizational champions" who are value driven, and the value that drives them is service; who stay close to the customer; who are sticklers for detail; who spend and (even overspend) on quality; who manage by walking around; and who make the typical employee a hero.

In a speech at the 1987 annual conference of the National Society of Patient Representatives held in Kansas City, Missouri, Sherman claimed that only uncommon leadership can save the health care industry. He described five characteristics:

- Uncommon leaders recognize who they are and what they are worth. They feel the greatness in their job and the capacity in themselves to fulfill this greatness. Their own self-esteem enables them to reach, stretch, and set elevating standards.
- Uncommon leaders understand the central truth of serving the customer. Sherman talks of Sam Walton, the richest man in the country, who spearheads Walmark Stores. Walton visits every one of his 700 stores annually. Walton's formula is simple: "Listen to

57

the customer. Believe what they say. Do what they tell you to do." Sherman adds that, historically, hospitals don't perform for their customers. They're concerned with making their customers conform to their policies.

- Uncommon leaders release the power in people. They know they can't do it all themselves. Believing that their people are their prime competitive advantage, they give credit.
- Uncommon leaders act like they own the place. The great architect Daniel Hudson Burnham said, "Make no small plans. Dream no small dreams!" Sherman adds, "If it is to be, it's up to me!"
- Uncommon leaders have one standard and one standard alone: *excellence*. Sherman says that nothing is wrong that can't be cured with a little leadership, with people who "grab for the gusto" and instead of feeling defeat, proclaim, "wait till tomorrow."

Organizational champions and uncommon leaders—that's what your strategy for service excellence needs. To achieve these ends, top management in health care needs to put into practice six principles that are critical if you are to drive toward excellence:

- Preach and lead with the vision.
- Practice what you preach and set the standard and the example.
- Hold people accountable.
- Empower your people: Support them. Ask, listen, act, inform, recognize, and reward.
- Take risks: Stick your neck out. Get off the dime.
- Go for the long haul, not the quick fix.

☐ Preach and Lead with the Vision

Managers become leaders by going beyond what is and seeking what might be. Your top management needs to define your vision of service excellence so that it's strong and motivating enough to propel your people and your organization toward excellence. A powerful vision that you chase ruthlessly inspires people. Without it, people get bogged down in detail and in the defeating aspect of day-to-day realities.

How do you begin to develop a powerful vision of service excellence? You start by imagining the perfect hospital environment from the patient's, doctor's, and employee's perspectives. How would you like to be treated as a patient, as a doctor, and as an employee? Project what an ideal workplace would be like. As an employee, what would make a day perfect, what surroundings would you like, how would you feel? As a guest, what would make the whole visit the least traumatic, the most comfortable? Once you have your own vision, you can share it with top management and ask what their personal vision of service excellence is. Then they in turn share their vision with those they lead and ask them to come up with visions of their own and then ask members of the work force for their vision.

Once your leadership and work force have each envisioned the reality they want for their organization, they must work toward forging a *common vision*. Ideally, the goal is what in business jargon is called an *aligned organization,* one in which the whole organization does all it can to achieve the common vision, to build a place where every manager, employee, and customer in the health care business would love to be.

Start by building into your organizational philosophy strong statements that communicate management's values, including excellence in service. Then, reiterate and reinforce this philosophy to drive behavior. Infuse your vision into the language your organization speaks. Figure 5-2 is an example of the Einstein Consulting Group's effort to apply this advice to its own rhetoric.

When you have a philosophy and value statement that illuminates your organization's vision, you then need to reinforce it when communicating your strategy for service excellence. Figure 5-3 is an example of a letter one CEO sent to all employees to kick off a strategy promoting service excellence.

Vision—without it, your people lack direction and inspiration. Your management team has to clarify their vision of service excellence and proclaim it across the land.

☐ Practice What You Preach

Once the vision is boldly communicated, management needs to translate this vision into specific standards that they set through their own behavior. When employees talk about administrators, common themes emerge. Many employees see their higher-ups as detached and out of touch with what's really happening on the front lines and concerned only with the bottom line. Administrators are often accused of exempting themselves from the standards they set for others, in other words, of failing to practice what they preach.

Administrative role modeling is the key to advancing the value of service excellence, to defusing excuses for resistance, and to motivating employees to do their part. Administrators can change the staff's perceptions by demonstrating personal commitment and by visibly showing the staff that no one, not even the bigwigs, is exempt from pressure to meet high standards of service excellence.

Exactly what should administrators do to set the example? Administrators need to put four behaviors into practice:

- Move close to customers.
- Model excellent customer relations skills.
- Model collegial support.
- Be visible.

Figure 5-2. Guiding Philosophy of the Einstein Consulting Group

Our company is set apart from others by our determination to turn a powerful vision into reality. We pride ourselves on having on our team *people who care about people* and who are inspired in their work by a desire to help others. In our health care work, we strive to improve for patients the quality, humanity, and dignity with which they are treated by health care employees and other care givers and to develop the skills, personal well-being, and harmonious relationships that are key to effectiveness and satisfaction in the stressful, important jobs of employees.

Our success as a company depends 100 percent on our people. We are committed to creating an environment that nurtures our employees so that we can fulfill our special mission.

In keeping with this philosophy, our job expectations are grounded in these values, which we reinforce repeatedly to drive us from our highly imperfect reality toward the ideals that we share.

1. *Empathy for Customers.* We are committed to giving the best customer service of any company in the world. Not some of the time, but all of the time. We are dedicated to addressing our customers' needs and will not compromise our ethics or integrity in the name of profit.
2. *Teamwork.* Our company relies on the initiative and involvement of everyone in innovation, problem solving, and execution of our individual responsibilities to improve our quality of work life and keep our promises to our customers. The job is too big to be done by some of us. We support each other and share our victories and rewards together.
3. *Excellence.* We are committed to quality. We care about what we do. To earn the respect and loyalty of our customers and to maintain our own energy and self-esteem, we need to pride ourselves on the excellence of our work. We identify, cultivate, train, reward, retain, and promote people who are committed to and effective in moving our organization forward.
4. *Dignity and Respect for the Individual.* We are committed to the importance of every employee. We believe in minimizing the distinctions and privileges of rank, treating every individual with respect and dignity, providing growth opportunities for every person, and sharing with every person the rewards of success.

It's an adventure, and we're in it together.

Figure 5-3. Letter Expressing Management Commitment

Dear Staff,

Next week, you'll be asked to attend your first experience with our new guest relations strategy: HOSPITALity. I'd like to tell you my hopes for HOSPITALity and why its success is so important to our hospital.

As I see it, the pressures on hospitals and on our hospital in particular are greater than ever. New government reimbursement arrangements have led to a revolution in how hospitals deliver services. We're seeing the results already: shorter lengths of stay per patient, sicker patients, cost cutting, reduced staffing, empty beds, insecurity, and competition among hospitals to make their facility the hospital of choice.

We're doing a great deal to maintain morale and also to compete effectively so we not only survive, but *thrive*. We're strengthening programs, adding new ones, publicizing services more aggressively, developing creative business arrangements, and in other ways, reaching out to our community. HOSPITALity reflects the role *every one of us* can play as individuals to help our hospital deliver true quality care that we can all be proud of and to strengthen our reputation and thus be the hospital of choice for our community.

I'm excited about HOSPITALity because I strongly believe we can become *distinctive* and *famous* for our HOSPITALity. After all, we're already good. With a little extra effort, I believe we can give every patient the excellent care and dignity they deserve. And this will attract people to our hospital better than anything else could. So, I'm hopeful and excited on the one hand.

On the other hand, I recognize that every one of you is working harder and is under more pressure than ever. This makes it difficult to extend yourself to people consistently. I realize that, and I know it's a lot to ask.

I'm placing a top priority on HOSPITALity now because of the pressures we're all feeling. We need each other more than ever. There's such a danger nowadays that the emphasis on the bottom line will overwhelm the real reason our hospital exists.

This is no time to minimize the importance of the human ingredient. This is a time when we need more than ever to protect the humanity we've always demonstrated proudly.

Every day, I see your hard work and determination to deliver top-notch services. I'm asking you to stretch on the human ingredient as well. We can help each other cushion the stresses of the times. We can impress our patients and visitors with not only our technical competence, but also our human generosity. I know we can make this hospital work for everyone.

Thank you for all you're doing.

Sincerely,
Helen Honcho

Move Close to Customers

If your management calls for an organizationwide priority on customer satisfaction, then management too needs to show attention
and concern for customers. How can management do this? They can
do it by taking personal steps to understand customer needs and
perceptions and by installing systems that identify customer needs
and invite complaints.

For example, administrators can dare to call on at least one patient,
one doctor, and one employee every working day. Not only will this
action build goodwill, it will also create a direct feedback channel
between you and customers, who are the end-users of the system
you're spearheading. Such feedback is the most powerful information
source you could ever have. Going to your customers shows your
employees and your customers that you care about the people on the
other end of your services.

Model Excellent Customer Relations Skills

Employees expect administrators to be role models and standard
setters in interactions with employees, patients, visitors, and doctors; and they're right to expect this. Management's behavior is an
opportunity to reinforce the behavior they want to see throughout the
organization. Also, accusations of hypocrisy and double standards
fade.

When Marsha Kurman of the Einstein Consulting Group asked
employees what administrative behaviors matter the most to them,
they most often cited behavior in public areas. Kurman says, "Administrators first need to become more visible and outgoing in these
public areas, in hallways, elevators, lobbies, the cafeteria. The key
here is to turn up the volume on their customer relations behavior. If
administrators do this just during their forays into public areas, they
can alter their image quite significantly." Your strategy for service
excellence should inspire employees to extend themselves to other
people in all work situations, no matter what their mood, and
especially in public areas where the atmosphere of the organization is
communicated.

Some administrators say that they want to be great role models but
lack the natural personality. Behaviors that result from feeling
awkward and uncomfortable in everyday workplace social situations
are seen by many employees as aloof, distant, indifferent, or uncaring.
Quiet administrators who visit a nursing unit and say little are
thought to be scrutinizing everything with a critical eye.

Administrators must stop using shyness or personality as an

excuse. After all, you wouldn't accept that excuse from front-line employees. Administrators can be shy, but they need to develop their own style of connecting to people positively and communicating friendliness, concern, and caring.

Administrators can use the following three-step, no-fail *image builder:*

- Make eye contact.
- Smile as you pass by.
- Occasionally say, "Hi, how's it going?"

Try the following suggestions from Marsha Kurman to move closer to your customers:

- *In the cafeteria:* your many options range from low risk to gutsy:
  —Eat in the employee cafeteria—more than once or twice.
  —If you feel awkward there, invite a colleague; another administrator is fine.
  —Make a decision to make eye contact with people and say hello, and then do it. You don't need to get into conversation.
  —Invite employees to eat with you. If you see people you know by name, ask them to join you.
  —If your awkwardness comes from worrying that the employee feels awkward, ease the tension by saying, "I want to get in touch with people here more than I've been. Yet, I feel awkward about it."
  —If you don't know people's names, pick out a person or two and say, "Hi, my name is _____. I'm an administrator here, and I don't believe we've met. There are so many people here I don't know. I want to change that. Would you like to join me for lunch?"
  —Invite yourself to join employees at their table. "Hi, I'm _____, an administrator here. If I wouldn't be interrupting too much, I'd like to join you for lunch. Would you mind?" For the first attempt, perhaps join an individual eating alone.
- *In elevators:*
  —Make eye contact and just say "hello."
  —Offer to push floor buttons for people.
  —Help the transporter with patients in wheelchairs or on stretchers. Open doors, for example. It's a friendly act, and shows teamwork.
  —Introduce yourself: "Hi, I'm _____. I don't believe we've met."
  —Make small talk: "How do you like this weather?" "I bet you have a busy day ahead of you." "How's our hospital treating you

lately?" "I see you work in the Dietary Department. How's it going?"
- *In hallways:*
  —The single most noticeable and important behavior is to establish eye contact, smile, and say "hello" to employees, patients,
  and visitors as you walk along instead of being withdrawn into
  your thoughts about your next meeting or that phone call you
  have to make.
  —Walk at a moderate pace so you don't appear too busy to notice
  the human beings along the way. Don't read memos and papers
  you're carrying.
  —Call people by name when you know them. A simple "Hello,
  Jim" suffices.

In quick interactions with employees, administrators can show
recognition and appreciation for customer relations behavior by
sharing a compliment. For example: "I've heard good things about the
burn unit. A woman wrote the other day about how pleased she was
with the way you folks handled her son. I think it was a Mrs. Jones."

Employees want, need, and deserve to see administrators extend
excellent customer relations. Administrators need to find ways, in
their own style, to connect to their employees and model positive
customer relations toward all guests. Doing this may mean changing,
but administrators ask that of employees all the time. Administrators
need to assess their own style, get feedback from coworkers, and
experiment with concrete improvements. The push for service
excellence that is reflected in nitty-gritty behaviors is everybody's job,
and administrators set the pace.

Model Collegial Support

Another administrative role that gets at best scant attention has to do
with the exchange of mutual support among the administrators
themselves. Few administrators are truly aware of their subordinates'
perception of top-level management as a group. For example:

> "They just go about their business, rushing around, sitting
> in meetings, solving problems, handling crises, prodding
> people to do their jobs, getting to the bottom of things."

or

> "Up there, one hand doesn't know what the other hand is
> doing. They don't know which end is up on the administra-
> tive floor!"

Would any administrator's heart be warmed by these employee perceptions? Would any administrator feel that these perceptions are "fair"?

Administrators endure tremendous stress because they are responsible for patients' experiences, the quality of life of the work force, and the organization's financial viability. To work successfully in a stressful environment, administrators need to support one another. They should not one-up one another, put one another down, or ignore one another's accomplishments. When they show a lack of mutual support, employees see it, lose confidence, and also follow suit in their behavior toward their own peers.

More than ever, administrators, like other employees, need the support of the entire organization. Begin by supporting one another. Administrators need to take active steps to develop their own image as strong, productive, and caring individuals engaged in a *team effort* to make the organization a place that works for everyone.

Here are some suggestions for developing support:

- Confront administrators who finger-point at one another. Expect your team to help and support one another. View every person's accomplishment as a team accomplishment and every problem as a team problem.
- Discuss how to handle situations in which one administrator gripes to another about a third person. Set a norm that requires confronting the person involved, instead of venting to a third party and feeding the behind-the-back grapevine.
- Practice delivering bad news to department heads without blaming another administrator. Proclaim the importance of "keeping the faith," and explore together ways to accomplish this when the going gets tough.
- Have administrators be role models of teamwork, mutual interchange, and information sharing by attending one another's meetings with department heads and employee groups.

Administrators need to market one another. Everyone wins when administrators promote one another, show respect, and acknowledge one another publicly as effective, accomplished leaders worthy of employee and patient trust. This mutual support among colleagues is inspirational for employees to see. It fuels the concept of service excellence and builds confidence in management.

Be Visible

A contemporary management commandment proclaimed by Tom

Peters is to "manage by wandering around (MBWA)." On the one hand, employees need to know who their leaders are, need to see them in action, and need to observe their interest in front-line people and their problems. On the other hand, administrators need to touch base with the operational realities and take the pulse of their employees.

However, just getting out of the boardroom and office and strolling around the workplace isn't enough. What goes on during that walking-around time can make or break the practice. Here are guidelines on what to do when you visit units and departments:

- Talk to people: "How are things going today?"
- Find out when most employees take their breaks or when the slower, calmer times are and visit then so that you're less intrusive. Tell the nurse manager or department head that you'd like to visit just to say hello and talk to people. Let people expect you.
- If you're uncomfortable, buddy up with a colleague who's good at this. One hospital formalized this type of visit as *walking-around training,* so that every administrator would be good at it and less hesitant to do it.
- *At the very least,* be sure to:
  —Smile.
  —Make eye contact.
  —Give your name.
  —Use the other person's name. If you don't know the name, ask it, and then use it.
  —Inquire about the employee personally, their work, their department, their life outside of work.

As you walk around, keep the following *don'ts* in mind:

- Don't tell anyone to do anything.
- Don't criticize anything. If you see a problem, address it through the proper channels later.
- Don't be a spy or judge.
- Don't be anything but happy. If you look concerned, employees will think you're concerned with the health of the organization, and they'll lose faith, or they'll take it personally and feel judged and paranoid.
- Don't miss anyone. Ask about the people who aren't around and say you're sorry you missed them.
- Don't be distracted. Listen to what people say, and the next time you see them, try to comment about what they said.

Most administrators want to increase their visibility, but they don't seem to get around to it. Their only hope, many claim, is to develop a schedule for wandering around in a time-limited way, to in effect make *short* excursions designed to increase their visibility. The key is to stick to this decision religiously because visibility is a priority and should not be the first activity to be eliminated when other demands arise. The following are tried-and-true methods for achieving administrative visibility:

- *Surprise welcome.* Administrators stand at a main entrance to the hospital for 30 minutes a day for one week and greet and introduce themselves to employees, visitors, and doctors. This welcoming activity should be done at different entrances at peak times of day so that the administrator can meet as many different people as possible. Administrators need to speak only briefly to each person: "Good morning. I'm not sure we've met. My name is Lee Weston. I'm an administrator. And you, where do you work? Very nice meeting you. Have a nice day."
- *Administrative grand rounds.* Employees often say that administration is out of touch with the real life on patient floors. Administrators can make rounds, visiting different units and work areas, greeting employees, introducing themselves, asking how things are going, and showing an interest in learning what different jobs are like. One idea that works well is to have a different administrator "on call" each week: this administrator makes daily rounds to a sampling of units and departments and talks with staff and patients.
- *Administrators as tray delivery squad.* To get to know about people's jobs and to touch base with patients, administrators can deliver food trays to patients for 30 minutes each week or two. This way they can spend a few minutes with each patient, introducing themselves and asking, "How have we been treating you?" Then the administrator should provide feedback to staff on any praise or problems mentioned by patients. Perhaps the administrator can write a positive piece for the employee newsletter based on the experience.

☐ Hold People Accountable

How accountable should your administrators be for employee and customer relations? Figure 5-4 shows a continuum of accountability. Consider your own position on the continuum.

Some people whose ratings fall toward the left of the continuum claim that administrators are just too busy and too far from the action

Figure 5-4. Accountability Continuum

Bad	Poor	Fair	Average	Good	Excellent
1	2	3	4	5	6

Administrators have little direct contact with either patients or employees and therefore cannot be held responsible for service excellence and customer relations. Administrators should have only a minor role in customer relations. The emphasis should be placed on those who are most accountable: the middle managers and supervisors.	Employees look to administrators as role models and standard setters. Administrators establish the culture regarding service excellence and customer relations. Because administrators are ultimately accountable, they should play a prominent role in the strategy for service excellence.

to be held responsible for the behavior of employees they don't even see. Others contend that administrators are responsible and accountable for employee behavior because they set standards in the first place and control consequences by deciding which behavior to reward and tolerate.

Unless you consider your administrators accountable, you're in an unworkable bind. Administrators, consciously or unconsciously, set the tone and standards for employee behavior. Employees watch administrative behavior and listen to their rhetoric. If the administrator does not insist on excellent service, employees get the message.

Administrators are bigger than life to employees. Their behaviors are watched and talked about. They set expectations as well as the tone and culture of the organization. They set up the internal accountability mechanisms. They set the rules and establish the systems. If a rude person is allowed to be rude year after year, how can you not point to administrative tolerance as the source of the unenforced standards? To escape the reality of administrative accountability is to negate the tremendous power of authority figures.

If your organization's strategy is aimed at service excellence, administrators have to pay determined attention to accountability. Specifically, they need to shape middle-management behavior so that the internal accountability mechanisms of the organization, the middle managers, internalize higher standards and engage in behavior that supports, enforces, and reinforces this behavior throughout the work force. The top people have to hold the middle people accountable, or else the middle people don't hold the front-line people accountable.

Consider an example from the airline industry. Under President Jan Carlzon, Scandinavian Airlines went from an $8 million loss in 1981 to a $71 million profit in less than a year. Carlzon's strategy was to transform the organization's focus from its internal production capabilities to an obsession with customer needs and desires. The company emphasized high standards of courtesy and service during every flight and in all peripheral services related to travel.

After a tremendous success, standards at Scandinavian Airlines started to slide. Planes started being late, employees were less cheerful, and service in general seemed to be getting sloppy. To try to learn what was wrong, Scandinavian Airlines conducted an organizational critique. They concluded that the quick change, with its emphasis on closeness to the customer, had bypassed middle management. Front-line people got more attention and rewards and more authority and resources to solve problems. Because middle managers felt left out, they resisted the changes. They continued to defend their own turf and operate according to their own individual ideas. This tug-of-war between top management's stated values and middle-management's ideas created a front-line motivation problem.

The example of the problems at Scandinavian Airlines shows that top management needs to:

- Consider carefully the middle manager's role in service excellence.
- Set explicit expectations for middle managers.
- Communicate these expectations to the middle managers.
- Show they mean business by monitoring middle-management performance and enforcing and reinforcing the expectations set.

Many top executives assume that middle managers know what to do. Perhaps that's true when it comes to their overall role. However, based on experiences with hospital middle managers across the country, it is most certainly not so with service excellence. Some middle managers consider service excellence peripheral, less important than the task specialties they hired people to perform. Others have long had problems with rude employees and have made excuses for not handling the problem: "there are always a few bad apples" or "you can't win 'em all" or "he's been here for so many years that it's too late now." The thought of raising standards and enforcing them is seen as just another pressure that will go away if it is ignored. Still others perceive no blatant problems in their departments, and so they feel strongly that they needn't do anything about service excellence. They've become accustomed to mediocrity, or in many cases, don't recognize the missed opportunities for their people to excel and impress their customers.

As a result, if top management is really serious about achieving service excellence, it must set new and serious expectations for middle management. Preferably these expectations will apply systemwide to all employees.

Following are some expectations for middle managers:

- Exemplify excellent customer relations in interactions with patients, visitors, doctors, and employees, and serve as a positive role model.
- Develop for or with every subordinate job-specific expectations that lead the employee toward service excellence.
- Hold regular meetings with subordinates to keep them informed of hospitalwide issues, events, and priorities and to identify and solve departmental problems.
- Monitor customer relations behavior: ask about it, comment on it, reinforce it, and reiterate its importance.
- Confront employees who violate customer relations expectations. Use the disciplinary process to counsel, coach, and, when necessary, terminate. Do not tolerate mediocrity.
- Develop and sustain open lines of communication with employees. Listen to employee concerns and respond in a timely, caring fashion.

Top management must hold department heads accountable for excellent service within their departments, or gradually service standards evaporate. Yes, I'm advocating finger pointing. In the face of complaints about rudeness of front-line employees, administration should investigate and hold the department heads accountable for the behavior of the people in their department. Incidents cannot be allowed to pass unnoticed.

☐ Empower Your People

Administrative behavior is mirrored at every level. If administrators support and empower their people, then other people follow their lead. If you think this statement is only rhetoric, let's look a little more deeply at the way administrators use their *power.*

Figure 5-5 shows the traditional structure of most organizations. The smallest number of people are at the top and have the most power. The people below are there to empower the people above, to serve needs as the people higher up see fit.

This structure is entirely inappropriate for service organizations. An organization intent on service excellence should turn this power hierarchy upside down: it should invert the traditional pyramid structure (figure 5-6).

Figure 5-5. Traditional Structure of Most Organizations

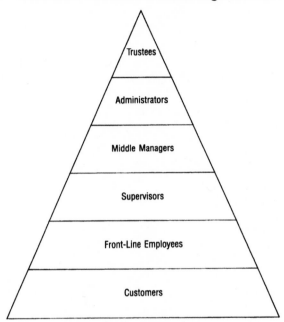

With this inverted-pyramid model, the customer's needs reign supreme. Your job as a manager is to *help your people to serve their customers.* The manager's role is to empower others, not to be empowered by them. Every layer of people below the customer is there to serve the needs of the people above. In this light, the administrator's job is to empower and support the department heads (and doctors) so that the department heads can support the supervisors, who can support the front-line employees, who can serve the customers.

Health care people have never understood this inverted pyramid. In fact, they have had it backward for a long time. In a structure geared to service excellence, the manager's role, according to Katie Buckley of the Einstein Consulting Group, is "to empower your people by motivating, encouraging, helping them do their all, and believing in them. When you're in the presence of a powerful person, you feel expanded. They aren't there to impress you by throwing their weight around. They're there to concentrate on you, to help you do all you can do. In turn, you do that for the customer."

The inverted-pyramid model has great implications for the administrator's role in service excellence. Administrators can empower their employees through effective use of support systems, communication and information, and recognition and reward.

Figure 5-6. Structure of an Organization Intent on Service Excellence

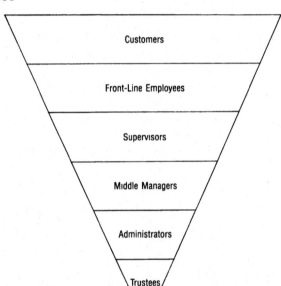

Empowerment through Support Systems

Once you've generated a powerful vision of service excellence, you need to take a hard, analytical look at where you and your organization are now. Given a clear picture of the discrepancies between vision and reality, administrators then need to look at what *they* themselves can do to enable their employees to better serve their customers.

In order for department heads to be responsive and helpful to their employees, administration needs to be responsive and helpful to department heads. Administrators can and should involve middle managers in developing concrete action plans for improving service, including goal setting with individuals, skill-building plans, periodic campaigns, and special events.

Employees also need to know that administrators are doing what they can to identify and solve problems that interfere with great service. Such problems include, for example, poor signage, a scarcity of wheelchairs in key areas, poor scheduling systems that produce long waits for patients, and broken phones.

To succeed with service excellence in the long run, management has to establish support systems that give employees the power to serve the customer. Developing support systems for gathering input, solving problems, and keeping lines of communication open are the job of top management. Only managers have the clout to create such systems and to make them work for everyone's benefit.

Empowerment through Communication and Information

Administrators also need to keep employees and physicians informed if they expect commitment, dedication, and salesmindedness. Truth telling about the organization's goals, challenges, strengths, and problems helps people feel respected and builds an identity with the organization. Administrators must level with people and avoid the temptation to shelter or exaggerate. People were not born yesterday, and they deserve and want to know the realities. Left unknowing, they resist doing their best in making the organization successful.

Administrators have great powers to sustain communication if they choose to use these powers. If they don't, informal and less controlled systems take over, much to the administrator's chagrin.

Empowerment through Recognition and Reward

If administrators espouse the importance of service excellence, then they need to provide rewards for employee commitment, excellent behavior, and salesmindedness. Administrators have the clout to create reward systems. They need to recognize the power of symbols and make rewarding symbols, for example, perks, incentive pay, prizes, praise, certificates, or awards, contingent on customer relations performance and not just on productivity or effective execution of technical skills.

To spread the gospel of service excellence, make examples of exemplary performers. Create your heroes, your superstars, by:

- Finding your best people
- Putting them on a pedestal
- Rewarding them
- Communicating their accomplishments and rewards to the rest of the staff
- Creating more heroes through standard setting, coaching, and reward

□ Take Risks

Since opportunity and danger are inseparable, it is impossible to make a significant step forward without encoun-

tering danger; and obversely, the scent of danger should
alert us to the fact that we may have headed in the right
direction.

—James Lipton

For most health care organizations, advancement toward consistently
excellent service and an obsession with satisfying customers means
change, and change triggers severe allergic reactions in most organizations, especially in health care. An enhanced emphasis on customer
satisfaction, the concept of the patient as a customer, pressure on
employees to achieve customer satisfaction despite how hard they are
already working, all of these involve culture change and changed
behavior on the part of individuals.

To trigger such change, top management has to decide to change
the organization. It has to make daring decisions. It has to follow
through and not back off. It has to take *risks*.

In *Managerial Courage: Revitalizing Your Company without
Sacrificing Your Job* (New York City: John Wiley and Sons, 1986),
Harvey Hornstein said: "Managers become leaders by going beyond
what is . . . and seeking what might be. Leaders ask fundamental
questions about the appropriateness and effectiveness of established
practice. They jeopardize their own welfare, since they're rocking
everyone's boat. Managers who ascend the corporate ladder because
they're compromising, cautious, and conforming are essential to the
successful maintenance of day-to-day organizational functions. They
keep the system running smoothly and predictably. They become
leaders only if they find the courage to question the system and risk
shaking it up."

Consider the culture of health care organizations. The image of a
turtle comes to mind. Slow as the turtle is, it makes progress only
when it sticks its neck out. The same is true for health care
administrators.

Risk taking by top management is a necessity in launching and
supporting your strategy for service excellence. Administrators are
rarely popular when they press for higher standards. One reason is
that even they can't be sure that their best-laid plans will actually
work.

The key to success then is an experimenter's mind set. No recipe
guarantees service excellence. There's no such thing as a quick fix.
The best administrators can do is research the possibilities at each
juncture, follow hunches, build on successes, and learn from mistakes. If your administrative people don't want to make a move until
they have guarantees, they will sit forever on the dime and your

organization will stagnate as it pays lip service to service excellence.

Franklin Delano Roosevelt said it: "It is common sense to take a method and try it. If it fails, admit it frankly and try another. But above all, try something." Tom Peters: "Do it. Fix it. Try it." Your management team needs to count on failing a little. If they do, perhaps they will brace themselves to be more resilient in the inevitable stops and starts that are part of any forward movement.

☐ Go for the Long Haul, Not the Quick Fix

Don't start up unless you plan to follow up. Service excellence only works as a long-term business strategy, as a continuous thrust that drives your organization.

Don't let your organization start until it is committed to continue year after year. If your service excellence effort is short-lived, the frustrated employee who says "just another flash-in-the-pan" will be painfully correct and understandably resentful.

Set objectives and plan for the future. Don't undertake change just to keep up with the Joneses. Know why you're doing what you're doing, and set objectives in terms of quality, costs, and risks.

In your organization, is service excellence rhetoric or reality? Does a long-term commitment to service excellence show up in management's annual budget as an operating expense line item that continues year after year, like salaries? Or are expenditures for service excellence an afterthought?

At a 1985 Innovators Conference sponsored by the National Society of Patient Representatives, Ray Stone, director of consumer affairs for the Marriott Corporation, said, "Don't embark on a customer relations program that you personally are not going to back 100 percent, and with more than executive memos." He added these words of Flip Wilson: "Don't let your mouth write a check that your body can't cash."

Commit dollars to service excellence. It's not a frivolous expenditure; it's a crucial and astute investment in quality.

If top management develops myopia about the benefits of a continued service commitment, try some of the following methods:

- Call in an outside expert on customer relations to talk about the necessity of follow-through. An outsider can present the false starts other hospitals experienced when they let up on their efforts. An outsider does not have to mince words. Also, administrators are more likely to listen to an outside expert.
- Create a diagnostic tool that pushes your administration to look at

components of a long-range strategy and to identify the missing links. Sometimes they realize they'll lose the hard-won gains they've achieved if they don't continue to attack weaknesses.

- Interview patients, visitors, doctors, and employees. Ask them what's going well and what still needs to be improved. Then use the survey to show your administration that more work is needed.
- Scrutinize the patterns of complaints and customer satisfaction information identified by your patient representatives.
- Convene committees for discharge planning, risk management, quality assurance, utilization review, and so forth. Do the same with department heads of key service departments. Ask them to identify further needs. Use their identification of problems and needs as evidence that the job is not yet done.
- Interview your long-range planning and marketing people to see if service excellence and service values have become ingrained in the hospital culture. If not, get an influential administrator on your side, someone who realizes that the corporate culture needs to support standards for service excellence. Also, get the marketing department on your side by advocating that internal marketing is an inherent piece of the organization's marketing plan.
- Collect published material that discusses what makes a service excellence or guest relations strategy successful in the long run. Channel these to administrators through people who influence them.
- Convene a group of people who are opinion leaders in the organization. Use any of the preceding strategies to convince them of the need for follow-up. Then brainstorm with them about how to get the necessary support from top management.
- Develop an explicit, specific plan for follow-up. Perhaps, you can bring in a consultant to conduct a stock-taking retreat. Present your concrete plan to your management team. Administrators often resist follow-up because they can't visualize it.

Management philosophy and practices are a critical underpinning of your strategy for service excellence and are worth dwelling on upfront—before you find your edifice crumbling.

☐ Final Suggestions

Be aware that certain myths can doom a strategy for service excellence to failure. If you hear any of the following statements made in relation to your strategy, you're in trouble if you don't act appropriately:

- *"They either have it, or they don't!"* This statement is not true about leadership. When it comes to service excellence, administrative support and leadership is on a continuum. Administrators, like other real people, vary: some are supportive, some skeptical, others cynical, and many changeable in their views. Although their rhetoric is a prerequisite to launching your strategy, you can still succeed even if they aren't perfect role models or gung-ho enthusiasts of service excellence. In a persistent, carefully wrought strategy, peer pressure and upward pressure from your savvy front-line people can gradually shape and strengthen administrators' behavior.
- *"I can't confront my administrator."* When administrators' lack of commitment of resources is eroding your efforts, you have to confront them. Avoiding confrontations is a disease. Usually the middle-management people are the ones running with the service excellence ball, and some people at this level sometimes shy away from confronting higher-ups with problems and needs. This attitude is not surprising. However, if these accountable people don't confront, they lose too, because they stand by as their strategy for service excellence weakens and gradually dies. And they get the blame. Given the trade-offs, middle-management people who have a stake in and responsibility for service excellence should creatively and persistently confront (or bring in an outsider to play the "heavy" and confront) top management about what the organization needs to do to make its strategy for service excellence deliver the hoped-for results.
- *"Administrators are just too busy. We shouldn't bother them."* Administrators are indeed incredibly busy. However, service excellence only takes hold if it's an organizationwide priority. Delegating it entirely just doesn't work. Also, if service excellence does not gradually seep into the minds and hearts of top management, they will not think, feel, and act in ways that advance it.
- *"A nonsupportive CEO dooms our effort to failure."* Having a CEO who isn't around much or isn't articulate about or supportive of service excellence is unfortunate. However, you can still secure the support you need to succeed. The CEO is not necessarily the only key. When I talk about the administrators' role, I'm talking about *all* administrators, not just your CEO. Vice-presidents and others may assume overt responsibility for your corporate culture. If they wait for the guru at the top to say "go," they, and you, may just wait forever. In many organizations, lower-level administrators can and do take the service excellence ball and run with it. In fact, because they are closer to the operations of the hospital and considerably more available, having them as vigorous advocates for service

excellence makes good sense. The question really is this: Does your organization have a critical mass of administrative support and involvement from *influential* administrators, even if these people do not include the CEO?

At one hospital, the CEO was planning to retire in a year and had withdrawn from his formerly aggressive leadership role. Everyone talked about how the hospital was at a standstill until new leadership arrived. Finally, other administrators joined together to move the hospital forward.

Lower-level administrators may also be the key even if the CEO is a strong advocate of service excellence. At another hospital, the CEO was the only wonderful customer relations role model in the system. The associate administrators and vice-presidents didn't act supportive, and they just didn't manage their department heads for service excellence. The result was no advances in service excellence—none whatsoever.

Management philosophy and commitment set the stage and enable the key players—every employee and doctor—to move in the same direction: toward customer satisfaction. Starting with a vision of service excellence, the top brass and every other layer of managers and supervisors need to set the tone through their own behavior; to build responsive, user-friendly systems that enable care givers to serve their customers; to communicate openly to build understanding, commitment, and investment; and to enforce and reinforce inviolable high standards.

Without management commitment, your organization has a perceived leadership vacuum that leaves the care giver and the patient floundering. With management commitment, you have a value-driven organization that has strength, focus, and inspiration at the helm.

Accountability

- You interview and hire an extremely competent nurse with impressive credentials. After she's been on the job for a while, you see that she has quite an attitude problem. "I can't understand it," you wonder in dismay. "After all we went through to hire the best person."
- A maintenance worker sees a film on caring and customer relations and thinks, "That's nice. But what does it have to do with me?"
- Many people wonder why a notoriously rude employee who's been a blemish on your hospital's image is allowed to continue this behavior unchallenged.

Marsha Kurman of the Einstein Consulting Group cites these situations as typical symptoms that reveal gaps in an organization's accountability systems, gaps that impede the achievement of service excellence. These situations are not unusual in hospitals. They typify organizations with weak links in their strategies for service excellence. They also typify organizations that are usually disappointed in the results of their strategies.

Accountability systems cannot be neglected in your strategy for service excellence. In the situations mentioned earlier, training is not the answer. The groundwork for accountability needs to be laid in revised personnel practices before training can be effective. In the first situation, says Kurman, a nurse with an attitude problem was given the job because hiring practices targeted technical competence at the expense of customer relations skills. In the second example, the new-employee orientation process did not ensure that the maintenance worker understood his or her role in the strategy for service excellence. In the third example, a problem employee's continued rudeness, year after year, demoralized and angered coworkers and, no doubt, turned customers off. Personnel practices actually pulled the "teeth" out of the customer relations standards.

How well do your current personnel policies support service excellence? To find out, take the self-test in figure 6-1. If you are able to answer "yes" to every question, accountability systems that support your commitment to service excellence are in place. The more "no" answers, the more you need to do to strengthen accountability so that your strategy for service excellence is powerful and enduring.

☐ Personnel Practices

Can people get a better raise for being exemplary in customer relations? Will employees who violate customer relations expectations suffer any consequences? Will disciplinary actions on customer relations behavior stick? Without "teeth" in your strategy for service excellence, you run the risk that negativity and mediocrity will continue to be tolerated.

Managers and supervisors need to know that they have backup support if they confront customer relations offenders. They need to know that they are *expected* to hold employees accountable to high service standards and that the system will support them if they do. They also need help in learning how to use the disciplinary process on hard-to-define interpersonal behavior.

Revamp or strengthen your personnel policies and practices to give "teeth" to your strategy for service excellence. In developing a consistent systems approach, you should do the following:

- Create a systemwide policy for service excellence.
- Develop explicit expectations for employee behavior.
- Build service expectations into job descriptions.
- Build service dimensions into your performance appraisal process.
- Hire the right people in the first place.
- Get your new people off on the right foot through your new-employee orientation.
- Develop a formal commendation process.
- Educate your management personnel about how to use the system.

Figure 6-1. Self-Test: How Well Do Your Current Personnel Policies Support Customer Relations?

Current Personnel Policies and Customer Relations. Circle the appropriate answer. If all the answers are "yes," your policies provide support for your strategy for service excellence. "No" answers indicate areas that need improvement.

1. Does your hospital *require* specific customer relations behaviors toward patients, physicians, and fellow employees?   Yes   No

2. Are your supervisors explicitly expected to be role models of exemplary behavior toward customers?   Yes   No

3. Does evaluation of behavior toward customers affect employee pay increases or promotions?   Yes   No

4. Are employees absolutely clear about what's expected of them in terms of behavior toward customers?   Yes   No

5. Are required customer relations behaviors spelled out in job descriptions?   Yes   No

6. Does your performance appraisal system specifically include an evaluation of employee behavior toward customers?   Yes   No

7. Does your process for new-employee orientation highlight your organization's commitment to service excellence and clarify the role of every individual?   Yes   No

8. Do you hire service-oriented people in the first place?   Yes   No

9. Do your supervisors and management personnel enforce customer relations standards?   Yes   No

Total: ___   ___

Create a Policy for Service Excellence

By issuing an overall hospital policy on service excellence, you can establish, in one simple action, that service excellence is *an organizationwide priority and a job requirement.* Such a policy:

- Shows employees clearly that excellent customer relations behavior is required of everyone no matter what their job or status and forewarns employees that customer relations problems can result in disciplinary action.
- Strengthens the likelihood that disciplinary actions related to customer relations will stick. If an employee being disciplined

claims to be unaware of the importance of customer relations behavior, the existence of the policy, with documentation about its distribution, discredits this excuse.

Figure 6-2 is an example of a hospitalwide policy that includes behavioral expectations.

Figure 6-2. Example of a Customer Relations Policy

A. Purpose
This policy provides guidelines for attitudes and actions by employees and physicians on the staff that foster favorable relations between employees and patients, patients' families, visitors, fellow employees, and the medical staff.

B. Philosophy
At the Albert Einstein Medical Center, Northern Division, we recognize that a patient's recovery is aided by sympathetic surroundings and that admissions to our hospital are affected by interpersonal relationships and by the image that our hospital projects. Further, we place a high degree of importance on establishing and maintaining an atmosphere of friendliness, courtesy, and concern for each patient, visitor, doctor, and coworker so that all of these people have a favorable perception of and experience with our hospital.

C. Policy
It is the policy of Albert Einstein Medical Center, Northern Division, to encourage and expect each person connected with the Medical Center to at all times:
1. Be aware of and concerned about how his or her attitude and actions affect patients and other individuals, including coworker relations, within the institution
2. Demonstrate appropriate demeanor as described within this policy and as contained within the HOSPITALity "House Rules" (behavioral expectations)

D. Definitions
1. *Appropriate demeanor:* an attitude or action in interacting with others (fellow employees, medical staff, patients, patients' families, and visitors) that includes:
   a. Observance of the HOSPITALity "House Rules"
   b. Courtesy and politeness
   c. Friendliness
   d. Concern for the patient's well-being
   e. Sensitivity and prompt responsiveness to the patient's wants and needs
   f. Cooperation with and helpfulness to the patient, members of the patient's family, visitors, and coworkers
   g. Pride in self, profession, and the hospital
   h. Respect for other human beings

2. *Favorable patient perceptions:* a patient's favorable perception reflects the following:
   a. He or she is treated as a welcomed guest of our hospital.
   b. His or her care is provided with sensitivity and responsiveness.
   c. The staff is courteous, concerned, and professionally competent.
   d. Respect and cooperation exist between employees to ensure optimum patient care and support services.
   e. The environment is clean, quiet, comfortable, secure, and properly equipped.

(continued)

Figure 6-2. *(continued)*

E. Responsibilities

1. It is the responsibility of each employee and physician to:
   a. Ensure that his or her attitude and actions are at all times consistent with the standards as described within this policy and as contained in the HOSPITALity "House Rules."
   b. Remind a coworker when his or her attitude or actions are inconsistent with these standards.
   c. Compliment a coworker when his or her actions comply with this policy.
   d. Call instances of excellence or noncompliance to the attention of the appropriate supervisor or department head.

2. It is the responsibility of each department head and supervisor to:
   a. Ensure that each employee under his or her jurisdiction upholds these standards.
   b. Investigate reports of and document instances of violation of these standards and take appropriate corrective actions, especially when behavior is shown to repeatedly or seriously contravene the standards of demeanor described above. Such appropriate action may include counseling and other levels of discipline, including discharge.
   c. Commend an employee under his or her jurisdiction whose attitudes and actions consistently far exceed these standards. Such commendation should include the issuance of a letter of commendation for placement in the employee's personnel file.
   d. Evaluate an employee's compliance with these standards as part of conducting regularly scheduled and special performance evaluations.
   e. Bring to the attention of the appropriate supervisor or department head instances of demeanor contrary to or consistently far in excess of these standards by an employee under the jurisdiction of another supervisor or department head.

Develop Explicit Expectations for Employee Behavior

A generic set of behavioral expectations for all employees, regardless of position, tenure, or status, should be included in your policy for service excellence and should be proclaimed far and wide. Maybe the thought of having to spell out in no uncertain terms what constitutes courteous, compassionate, and respectful treatment of people is discouraging. However, in health care, service excellence involves far more than the popular view of courtesy as "niceness." It is more than just pasting a smile on your face. Is it any wonder then that hospitals without explicit behavioral expectations insult their employees who think that money, time, and attention are being spent on making them smile and be nice? Are accusations that customer relations workshops are "charm schools" really unwarranted when you don't detail the complex behavior involved in health care customer relations? After all, hospitals are not hotels, whose staff interact with largely happy people who've chosen to be where they are and who tend not to be fraught with anxiety and fear. The point is that you need to be specific about the intricacies of health care customer relations in order to move beyond "charm school" imagery and the hotel model.

Behavioral expectations can be established in two ways:

- You can develop expectations yourself by asking, "What should employees do to convey their compassion and respect to every one of our key customer groups?" Ask this question of patients as well as employees. Compile a list of behaviors. Narrow them down and consolidate them. Issue the narrowed-down list as generic expectations.
- Purchase a program from a consultant who knows hospitals. For instance, Einstein has developed 16 "House Rules" that more than 120 hospitals now use. Here are examples of these rules:
  —Help each other and help the patient.
  —Break the ice with people: smile, introduce yourself, call people by name.
  —When someone needs help, help the person or find someone who can.
  —Respond quickly. When people are worried or sick, every minute is an hour.

Build Expectations into Job Descriptions

To quickly instill customer relations into people's jobs, include statements describing customer relations expectations in their job descriptions. This action serves four purposes:

- Employees see that customer relations expectations are explicitly part of their jobs. When they look over their job descriptions for any reason, they are then reminded of the importance of customer relations.
- Employees know that an evaluation of their job performance will include a customer relations component because their job description indicates that providing excellent service to all the hospital's various customers is a function of their jobs.
- In disciplinary situations, the supervisor can show that the employee knew about customer relations requirements because "it's right there in the job description."
- Job applicants and new employees can be shown what is expected of them up front.

You can build customer relations into job descriptions by using broad, generic statements that apply to all employees or by developing job-specific statements:

- Broad generic statements are much easier to institute because they apply to every employee regardless of position. Here are examples:

—Generic job description statements for employees with supervisory or management responsibility (including administrators): "Exemplifies excellent customer relations toward patients, visitors, physicians, and coworkers; holds subordinates accountable for conformity to the 'House Rules.'"

—For nonsupervisory employees: "Exhibits excellent customer relations to patients, visitors, physicians, and coworkers; shows courtesy, compassion, and respect; conforms to the 'House Rules.'"

• Job-specific expectations take more work but are more likely to elicit the desired behavior. They spell out the unique opportunities for service excellence inherent in a particular position. The following job description statement is for an employee in the admissions office: "welcomes patients and visitors to the hospital and to the department; introduces self, calls guests by name, explains what patients and visitors can expect (their when's, why's, and how's); takes actions to make customers comfortable and to respond to their concerns."

Employees and their supervisors can work together to define these requirements, or you can involve your personnel or human resources people.

Build Customer Relations into Performance Appraisal Process

Customer relations behavior should be considered as a key component when employee behavior is evaluated. How such an evaluation is accomplished depends on your organization's performance appraisal system. Look at your system and figure out the best way to incorporate customer relations.

The four most common types of performance appraisal systems are those that focus on traits, on a person's major job requirements, on objectives for the year, and on performance standards.

Here are examples of each. Examine your system and look for the model most like yours. These models illustrate ways to build customer relations into all four types.

• If your performance appraisal system focuses on *traits*, you should include customer relations as a trait to be evaluated. If the system already has a trait called "attitude," replace it with "customer relations" or the name you're using for your program, for example, HOSPITALity at Einstein (figure 6-3).

• If your system focuses on *major job requirements* or *key tasks*,

Figure 6-3. Performance System Appraisal That Focuses on Traits

Performance Review	Albert Einstein Medical Center	Date:	Annual ( ) Probation ( ) Termination ( )
Name:	Title:	Dept.:	Special ( )

Instructions: You should comment on all factors: Circle appropriate numbers. You must comment on all ratings below 4 or above 7.

	Inadequate	Adequate	Satisfactory	Commendable	Outstanding
Job Knowledge: understanding of procedures, work methods, and techniques; effective utilization of resources	1 2 Comment:	3 4	5 6	7 8	9 10
Initiative: willingness to assume responsibilities; resourcefulness; creativity; meeting deadlines	1 2 Comment:	3 4	5 6	7 8	9 10
Judgment: logical decisions; intelligent application	1 2 Comment:	3 4	5 6	7 8	9 10
Hospitality: demeanor, courtesy, concern, politeness, "House Rules"	1 2 Comment:	3 4	5 6	7 8	9 10
Special Factor:	1 2 Comment:	3 4	5 6	7 8	9 10
Summary Rating: (The summary rating is not necessarily an average of the specific ratings.)	1 2 Comment:	3 4	5 6	7 8	9 10

Reprinted with permission of the Albert Einstein Medical Center, Northern Division include a customer relations statement (either generic or specific) as one of these tasks (figure 6-4). The statement can be the same as the one recommended for job descriptions discussed previously.

- If your system focuses on *objectives* for the year, provide supervisors with sample objective statements related to customer relations. You can use job description statements or more specific goal statements. The following are sample objectives for the year:
  —For a receptionist: "To welcome patients and visitors in a consistently friendly, cooperative, and helpful manner."
  —For a unit clerk: "To improve customer relations behavior toward doctors (greet them by name, move quickly to obtain their charts, and exhibit friendly, professional nonverbal behavior)."
- If you have a system focusing on *performance standards,* you must back up the series of dimensions, such as quality of work and attendance, with *standards* that define each possible rating. If you have such a system, include customer relations as a dimension and spell out standards related to it. Be careful to define *high* standards. Mediocre customer relations should be in the unacceptable category, because your standards should push people beyond mediocrity to excellence. Figure 6-5 shows an example of such a performance appraisal system used by Community Memorial Hospital in Toms River, New Jersey.

Hire the Right People in the First Place

Although selecting the right person for the job from a service excellence point of view has no scientific basis, you can hire better people by paying explicit attention to an applicant's interpersonal skills and philosophy. In "Customer Relations: The Personnel Angle" (*Personnel*, 1987 Sept., 64[9]:38-40), Marsha Kurman recommends these methods of improving screening practices:

- Make sure the person screening applicants, for example, your employment manager, personifies positive customer relations. The screener must be skilled, knowledgeable, and sensitive about customer relations and must be able to recognize customer relations skills and instincts in job applicants. The kind of person often hired as patient representative, patient advocate, guest relations coordinator, or employee relations director is the kind of person who should screen or help screen applicants, because these people can recognize the nuances in a person's style.
- Draw out an applicant's interpersonal skills and philosophy. For instance, ask open-ended questions about the applicant's previous job experience and listen for references to people skills and

Figure 6-4. Performance Appraisal System Focusing on Major Job Requirements

Rating Factors	Emp. Intl.	Performance Scale						
		Unacceptable	Far Below Requirements	Below Requirements	Meets Acceptable Requirements	Occasionally Exceeds Requirements	Regularly Exceeds Requirements	Far Exceeds Requirements
Brief description of major job requirements:								
Guest relations: Exemplifies high standards of hospitality in behavior toward patients, physicians, subordinates, and other coworkers. Holds subordinates accountable for conformity to the "House Rules."		Comments:						
Job Knowledge: Demonstrates knowledge of requirements and methods involved in doing the job.		Comments:						
Managerial skills (if applicable): Sets objectives and priorities, plans work effectively. Meets objectives within limits of time and cost. Delegates appropriately. Uses good judgment in decision making and problem solving.		Comments:						

situations. Examples of some questions to ask are:
— "What skills do you pride yourself on?"
— "What do you think it takes for a person to be successful in the job you're interviewing for?" (No matter what the position, you want all the people who work in your organization to be sensitive to other people.)
— "What in your last job did you enjoy?" (Look for malcontents.)
• Look for social skills and nonverbal presence:
— Does the applicant listen to you when you talk?
— Does the applicant make eye contact when meeting you and speaking to you?
— Does the applicant speak with feeling, empathy, and enthusiasm and not in a monotonous, flat tone?
• Ask the applicant to show his or her way of handling tough situations. For example, "If you saw a lost visitor in the hallway and you have a meeting to get to, what would you do?"

A most important part of the screening process is the interviewer's *mind set.* If you *look* for customer relations skills in a person, you'll be able to see what's there, and you can then hire the person who,

Figure 6-5. Part of a Performance Appraisal System That Focuses on Performance Standards

Performance Evaluation			
Employee:		Position title:	
Department:		Type of performance evaluation:	
Rating period: _____ to _____		[ ] 3 month [ ] 6 month [ ] annual	
Key Performance Factors	Rating		
	1	2	3
1. Hospitality			
2. Quality of work			
3. Quantity of work			
4. Cooperation			
5. Plans and organizes work			
6. Attendance			
Overall Performance Rating	1 Outstanding	2 Meets Requirements	3 Needs Improvement

(continued)

Figure 6-5. *(continued)*

Performance Factors	(1) Outstanding	(2) Meets Requirements	(3) Needs Improvement
1. Hospitality	Employee always follows "House Rules."	Employee always follows "House Rules."	Employee does not follow "House Rules."
	Supports the HOSPITALity program and encourages others to do the same.	Supports the HOSPITALity program.	Support of the HOSPITALity program is not always displayed.
	Serves as a role model to fellow employees by projecting an exceptional positive attitude.	Always displays a positive attitude.	Needs to put forth an extra effort to display a positive attitude.
2. Quality	Regardless of situation, always completes work assignment with exceptional accuracy.	Work completed is accurate and acceptable in all respects.	Most work completed is accurate, but some mistakes are discovered.
	Work usually exceeds standards and is thoroughly checked and needs no follow-up.	Employee conducts spot checks to ensure that work meets standards.	Employee does not always spot-check work to discover errors or problems and take corrective action.
	Work consistently brings praise for its high quality.	Work rarely needs follow-up.	Work needs frequent follow-up to ensure objectives, accuracy, and expectations.

Performance Standards Key

Reprinted with permission of Community Memorial Hospital, Toms River, New Jersey.

technical skills being equal to those of other candidates, excels in interpersonal skills.

Make sure all the people in your personnel area reflect your organization's value on service excellence. Applicants, like patients and visitors, spread the word to others about your institution. Do all you can to make sure that the word they spread is positive. Even if they don't get the job, they should leave feeling that your institution is a place in which they'd like to work. Leave them thinking "If I needed a hospital, I'd come here" and not "If their personnel office is any indication of what the rest of the place is like, I'll never be a patient there." The personnel office should reflect so well on your institution that good people want the job.

To check out your personnel department, evaluate it in terms of the following:

- Is your personnel staff role-modeling service excellence by being courteous, friendly, and responsive?
- Do staff greet applicants warmly and quickly and treat them as guests, not as intruders or strangers?
- Do office procedures show that the organization values service excellence?
- Is the personnel office a comfortable, attractive spot where applicants can complete their application and wait?
- Does someone provide applicants with coffee or tea and offer to hang up their coats?

During the hiring process, clarify that the purpose of probation is to assess not only technical skills, but also customer relations skills. Probation also gives the employee a chance to decide if your institution is for them, if their values and standards match yours. Make it clear that you will not negotiate about standards and that you want only people who can meet your standards fully. Mention that not every applicant may be comfortable with your organization's standards and ask the applicant to react to this.

Use the probationary period to test a person's interpersonal skills. If the person doesn't show the customer relations potential you expected, act quickly. Holding out for the right person is easier than hiring and keeping the wrong one and then being frustrated by their shortcomings forever after.

Get New People Off on the Right Foot

Your hospital has just hired some new employees. From day one, they must know the value you place on service excellence and the precise expectations you have for their behavior. Depending on osmosis to slowly take its course is a mistake.

Your new-employee orientation should communicate the difference between service excellence in your hospital and any other service settings in which the new employees may have previously worked. Before any negative proclivities of a new employee, such as inattentiveness, impatience, or indifference, are allowed to take hold in this new environment, set the record straight and start the new employee off on the right foot.

Chapter 6

In a more positive vein, new-employee orientation is a golden opportunity to convey the mission and value sacred in your organization's culture. In this orientation, you should:

- *Give the big picture about your organization, its mission, challenges, and strategies for success.* Explain how every employee is important to the organization's strategy for service excellence. Specifically, emphasize that every employee has customers. For some, the customer is the patient and the doctor. For others, the customer is another employee. So, everyone is the key to service excellence by either serving patients directly or serving people who do.
- *Encourage people to mix with one another. Structure orientation so that people get to know one another.* You are thus exemplifying the value you place on the human ingredient. A straight lecture hour after hour hardly reflects the importance you give to your people.
- *Set clear expectations about what constitutes excellent job performance.* Be behavioral, and avoid extensive talk about attitude. Your explanation of the generic expectations that every employee in your organization is expected to meet should be lively, anecdotal, and illustrative. Set high standards right off the bat, and communicate assertively that these standards are part of every person's job and are not guidelines or helpful hints.
- *Touch people's emotions.* Emphasize the point that whether at the bedside, in the laundry, or at a computer terminal, the primary concern of each employee is the patient. Sometimes you can use videos to communicate this message: for example, "You Make the Difference," "Not Just Another Day," and "You Are This Hospital" are available from the Einstein Consulting Group; and "Caring...It Makes a Difference" and "Sometimes . . . It's Harder to Care" are appropriate videos that are available from the American Hospital Association.
- *Give service excellence prominence during orientation* by:
  —Allocating time to service excellence in proportion to its value. How much of the orientation is spent on customer relations? 20 minutes? A full day? Do you leave it out if you're running late?
  —Positioning your service excellence component in prime time, and not as a filler.
  —Making sure that an advocate of service excellence conducts the session. The CEO, a gung-ho administrator, or a front-line worker all have natural credibility. Personnel and training professionals can also conduct this portion but only if they are effective communicators and believers.

—Following through after the initial component in orientation. For instance, two months after orientation, have an administrator reconvene new employees for breakfast to find out about their first months on the job. Other organizations have buddy systems: pairing an experienced, positive employee with a new employee.

Someone in top management should be part of new-employee orientations. If your top administrator doesn't show up reliably to speak to your new employees during orientation, change your method. Take the new employees en masse to his or her office. This action may make the administrator feel important and comfortable. Also, it gives new employees a first-hand opportunity to see the executive staff and office in operation.

Develop a Commendation Process

Consequences are a powerful influence over people's behavior. Too often, supervisors emphasize consequences for negative behavior but neglect positive consequences for positive behavior.

When a negative emphasis is allowed to prevail, your strategy for service excellence is tinged with a punitive, negative, watchdog overtone. Such a tone is not only demoralizing to employees, but it also fails to shape the behavior you want: it does not energize people or call attention to the people who shine.

To counteract this tendency toward negativism and to fuel your strategy for service excellence with energy, you must strengthen your organization's methods of focusing on the positive with praise, recognition, and appreciation. Consider using the following methods:

- *Formal use of your performance appraisal system.* Once you build customer relations into your performance appraisal system, use the system to formally reinforce positive behavior. Ideally, excellent customer relations can result in high ratings that translate into merit increases.
- *Verbal and written feedback.* Supervisors need to be encouraged to increase their *daily* use of verbal and written positive feedback to employees. For example: "I noticed you going out of your way to comfort that upset woman who was being admitted this morning. I saw you really focus on her, listen, show empathy, and do what you could to give her confidence in us here. Your customer relations skills were wonderful. I want you to know I admire it and appreciate what you did." No one can get too much praise, recognition, and appreciation. In fact, most people probably never get enough of it.

- *Recognition systems.* In addition to "Employees of the Year" or "Employees of the Month," consider methods that recognize *more* people *more* often. See chapter 12 on rewards and recognition for a smorgasbord of approaches.
- *Formal commendation system.* Most organizations have disciplinary documents as part of their personnel policies and procedures. However, the absence of a positive counterpart serves only to emphasize the negative. Institute a commendation form as a standard part of your personnel practices. Einstein uses a two-part form to reinforce the HOSPITALity priority (figure 6-6). This form is issued by supervisors. One copy is awarded to the employee, and the other copy is placed in the employee's personnel file as part of their permanent record.

Educate Management and Supervisory Personnel

Let's assume that you develop a stunning set of written policies and procedures that support service excellence and give your strategy some "teeth." None of these policies and procedures matters one iota

Figure 6-6. Sample of a Commendation Form

HOSPITALITY. COMMENDATION

Employee Name: Jeanne Martin

Department: Environmental Services

Situation Observed: The worried wife of a patient had become lost in the hospital.

Date: 12/18/85

Exemplary HOSPITALity Behavior: Jeanne took time out of a busy workday and walked the visitor up two flights of stairs to the room she was looking for, all the while being friendly and reassuring.

Statement of Appreciation: Jeanne's small but important act of compassion made me feel proud to work in the same hospital. I thank her not only on behalf of the visitor she helped, but also for making where I work a better place.

Katherine Zellerbach

Signed Katherine Zellerbach
Director of Environmental Services

Reprinted with permission of the Albert Einstein Healthcare Foundation, Philadelphia, Pennsylvania.

unless your supervisors and managers *use* them to hold people accountable.

Typically, a hospital's disciplinary process needs no modification to be applicable to customer relations. However, most supervisors need help using existing personnel practices and the disciplinary process to confront problems. Customer relations violations are hard to grasp, hard to describe behaviorally, and, therefore, hard to document effectively.

You must reeducate your managers and supervisor to use the improved system. Teach them the skills they need to hold employees accountable. To use the system properly, managers and supervisors need to:

- See themselves as role models.
- Commit themselves to upholding the organization's commitment to service excellence.
- Learn how to use feedback to shape and coach employees.
- Develop specific skills in confronting and counseling and in using disciplinary procedures for customer relations offenders.

Training sessions can help you demonstrate model behavior and give managers and supervisors substantial practice. However, learning to use these skills well is not easy. If you have in-house trainers who can help your managers master these skills, great. If not, spend the money to get outside help.

☐ Final Suggestions

The following suggestions will help you work on accountability:

- *Don't talk about attitude.* Instead, talk about behavior. Define for employees the behavior you want and set inspiringly high standards. People think they have good attitudes, and if you imply otherwise, they get defensive and accuse you of having an attitude problem yourself. You're at loggerheads because attitude is debatable, elusive, invisible, arguable. So let people keep whatever attitude they want; but demand and expect appropriate *behavior*, and define what that behavior is in no uncertain terms.
- *Mean what you say.* Devising elegant personnel practices is pointless unless you're going to inform people about them and enforce them. An excellent personnel policy that is not enforced is just another reflection of double standards and failure to follow through. In one large urban hospital, a top administrator's secretary,

Hilary, was notoriously rude to people. In an ambitious series of mandatory customer relations workshops, many employees resisted new high standards by pointing to Hilary. They said, "If you were serious about customer relations, Hilary wouldn't be here." They were right. You must confront such problem employees and coach and counsel them on how to change their behavior to relect service excellence. If they cannot meet your standards, you have to be ready to terminate their employment. However, if they do meet the challenge, you must be ready to reward them.

- *Have written job descriptions.* These descriptions should include performance expectations with regard to customer relations that are inherent in, and not peripheral to, the job. If you don't have written job descriptions, then how are people supposed to know what's part of their jobs? Of course, most people do know without your telling them. However, problem employees can use a lack of explicitness as an excuse for inappropriate behavior, asking, "Where's it written?"

Accountability, or the lack of it, can make or break your strategy for service excellence. As is true in most organizational change strategies, policies and practices require reexamination and revision. Although this process may be time consuming and cumbersome, the results more than justify the effort. Hiring customer-oriented people prevents later regrets and the ongoing need for excessive retraining. Policies and practices that clearly hold managers and staff accountable for achieving your higher standards make success achievable in the long run. And finally, you have to keep stressing and reinforcing the message that all employees are accountable for service excellence.

□ **Chapter 7**

Input and Evaluation

How can you measure the effectiveness of your strategy for service excellence? How can your organization obtain information from its key customer groups so that it can be self-renewing and self-improving? Traditionally, systems for obtaining systematic and regular information from customers have not been at the top of most organizations' priority lists. Yet, staying close to your customers is a first step toward meeting your customers' needs. Does your organization gauge customer satisfaction by more than the feelings and opinions of success or failure on the part of management and staff, or do you use a single global (and therefore not too informative) indicator like census?

Specific systematic sources of information from each key customer group, sources that rely on a mix of quantitative and qualitative methods, are needed to assess and improve your entire strategy for service excellence. These old adages speak volumes:

- Until you measure, you don't control.
- People respect what management inspects.
- You can't manage it unless you measure it.
- You can't tell if you're winning without a score.

You need to ask yourself the following questions:

- Does your organization currently assess the satisfaction of its:
  —Patients?
  —Visitors?

—Physicians?
—Employees?
- What exactly are your current assessment methods, both formal and informal?
- How helpful are your current methods?
- To what extent are results effectively fed to people who can act on them to improve your organization?
- To improve your systems for assessing satisfaction, you need to focus on:
  —Which priorities?
  —Which customer groups?
  —Which evaluation systems or methods?

☐ What to Measure

Measure customer perceptions along key service dimensions and dig for complaints. Don't forget to measure the perceptions and complaints of all customer groups: patients, visitors, physicians, employees, and third-party payers.

Perceptions

Start with perceptions. If your organization is typical, a central objective of your strategy for service excellence is to improve customer *perceptions* of the care, courtesy, compassion, and respect employees extend to them. The emphasis here is on the word *perceptions*, not actual behavior. Of course, changed behavior by employees is what causes changed perceptions by the customer. However, measuring changed behavior directly is too difficult. Yes, you can use observation techniques to count the frequency of certain behaviors. You can station observers in the admissions waiting area and have them watch admissions staff and count the number of smiles, words of concern, or uses of a person's name; but such observational techniques are cumbersome and time consuming. Not only that, but even if these behaviors were found to increase, your strategy has not reaped the expected results if patients and visitors don't perceive the improvement. If your strategy for service excellence measurably improves guest perceptions of your organization's staff, care, and services, then you have an indicator of success, a positive concrete result.

Complaints

As has been said elsewhere in this book, you should invite complaints. In fact, beg and plead with your customers to voice their complaints to you. According to Arlene Malech, TARP: Technical Assistance Research Project, properly handled complaints can build customer loyalty. Look at these statistics:

- 84 percent remain loyal (buy again) if you solve a complaint quickly.
- 54 percent remain loyal if the complaint is resolved—even if it takes some time.
- 19 percent remain loyal after they complain and the concern is not resolved.
- 9 percent remain loyal after identifying a problem and not complaining about it.

Complaints are a tremendous opportunity, a second chance to make things go right. Patient representatives have recognized this opportunity for years. Instead of discouraging complaints, your systems of input and evaluation (including but not limited to your patient representatives) should encourage your customers to share their frustrations, dissatisfaction, resentments, and suggestions.

Perhaps you think that if you invite more complaints and get them, the powers that be in your organization will conclude that your strategy for service excellence is failing. Convince them otherwise. An increase in complaints is rarely a sign of failure just as a reduction in complaints does not signal success. The number of complaints is largely a function of the organization's openness to complaints and to improving itself.

Some hospital people only begin encouraging complaints once they understand the positive value of complaints in their striving for service excellence. After they have instituted a strategy for service excellence, they experience an initial increase in complaints as a result of increasing staff openness and responsiveness.

Although the frequency of complaints increases, in the long run the ratio of complaints to appreciative comments decreases. If your strategy for service excellence is working, the content of the complaints will shift from complaints about rudeness to complaints about room temperature, an insufficient variety of video movies, and too infrequent visits by the energetic volunteer with the craft cart.

□ Methods Abound

After you assess your current methods for input and evaluation, decide whether they adequately accomplish their purposes in an efficient manner. If not, consider developing, once and for all, a sound, systematic, streamlined evaluation strategy that taps the perceptions of every one of your key customer groups.

Many approaches—some do-it-yourself, some involving outside resources—are available. Following are various methods you can use for each of your key customer groups:

Measuring Patient Satisfaction

By measuring patient satisfaction, you can:

- Measure the effects of your strategy for service excellence on customer perceptions of employee behavior.
- Identify positive results that you can use to acknowledge people and celebrate achievements.
- Identify negative results and complaints that give you an informed chance to make improvements in specific facets of your organization and strengthen your overall strategy.
- Obtain straight-from-the-source data that you can feed back to staff to help them stay close to their customers.

Most hospitals already have *live* data collectors—their patient representatives. Many patient representatives already have in operation excellent systems for tracking complaints and identifying patterns that merit attention.

You should enlist patient representatives in your efforts to measure customer satisfaction. In addition, you can use any one or all of the following methods: patient satisfaction surveys, postdischarge interviews, and patient focus groups.

Patient Satisfaction Survey

Perhaps your hospital already surveys patients before and after discharge. This kind of survey may be a good, and perhaps the best, tool for measuring customer perceptions of staff behavior if it:

- Contains items or dimensions specific to customer relations, for example, courtesy, concern, attention, responsiveness, explanations, and friendliness
- Yields an ample response (10 percent is low, 40 percent is hard to believe, and 30 percent is good and achievable)
- Is easy to fill out and understandable to users
- Is designed to ask openly for opinions, instead of being a public relations ploy designed with smiling faces and hype that influence the respondent
- Asks about specific areas (for example, nursing courtesy) so that

you can tell what it means and act on it

Most hospitals that use surveys mail the survey to discharged patients within a week of their discharge. When the returns are in, the data are processed, and the results are disseminated to the appropriate people and departments by the patient representatives, directors of marketing, or quality assurance or risk management people who manage the patient satisfaction measurement function.

To make the most of a survey like the one in figure 7-1, analyze the percentage of positive responses to get base-line information *before* you institute your strategy for service excellence. Then repeat the process at least quarterly to see how you're doing.

The survey results need to be summarized and circulated to people who are close to the action and who can act on the results. Carefully analyze the specific items that address service excellence. Also, analyze results by shift and by unit so that the results can be provided as feedback to specific shifts, units, and departments.

If you don't already have a patient satisfaction survey or if you don't have anyone on staff who is able to develop one, consider buying a standard instrument or one designed especially for your organization. Some good, relatively inexpensive patient satisfaction surveys and services are available from these people:

- Press Ganey Associates, Irwin Press, president, P.O. Box 1064, Notre Dame, Indiana 46556, 219/232-3387
- The "PERC System," Health Surveys and Marketing, Columbia, Maryland, Ellen Tobin, president, 301/730-2195
- The National Society of Patient Representatives, 840 N. Lake Shore Drive, Chicago, Illinois 60611, 312/280-6000

Postdischarge Interviews

A wonderful source of feedback, postdischarge interviews involve talking to randomly selected patients or to all former patients within two weeks of discharge. These interviews can yield quantifiable data, although qualitative results are tremendously helpful as well.

At Aultman Hospital, in Canton, Ohio, a patient callback system gives the Emergency Department valuable information about patients' experiences. According to the September 1986 issue of the newsletter *Convenience Care Update* (published by United Communications), two full-time registered nurses with emergency nursing experience share the position of 40-hour-per-week telephone communicator. A nurse phones patients 48 to 72 hours after their emergency department visit, asks questions from a carefully developed form, and

Figure 7-1. Example of a Postdischarge Patient Satisfaction Survey

YOUR COMMENTS WILL HELP US TO IMPROVE.

Please rate our care and services as you perceived them during your stay at

Your Admission:

	Yes	No
01 Through admission office	[ ]	[ ]
02 Through emergency unit	[ ]	[ ]

	Exc.	Good	Fair	Poor
03 Prompt	[ ]	[ ]	[ ]	[ ]
04 Courteous	[ ]	[ ]	[ ]	[ ]
05 Efficient	[ ]	[ ]	[ ]	[ ]
06 Room available promptly				
07 Explanation of financial information	[ ]	[ ]	[ ]	[ ]
	1	2	3	4

Comments

Preadmission Testing:

	Exc.	Good	Fair	Poor
08 Prompt	[ ]	[ ]	[ ]	[ ]
04 Courteous	[ ]	[ ]	[ ]	[ ]
05 Efficient	[ ]	[ ]	[ ]	[ ]
	1	2	3	4

Comments

Your Meals:

	Yes	No
23 Were you visited by a dietitian?	[ ]	[ ]
24 Were you on a special diet?	[ ]	[ ]
	1	2

	Exc.	Good	Fair	Poor
25 Tasty and appetizing	[ ]	[ ]	[ ]	[ ]
26 Proper temperature				
27 Efficient and courteous				

Comments

Other Services:

	Exc.	Good	Fair	Poor	No contact
28 X ray	[ ]	[ ]	[ ]	[ ]	[ ]
29 Laboratory	[ ]	[ ]	[ ]	[ ]	[ ]
30 Electrocardiography	[ ]	[ ]	[ ]	[ ]	[ ]
31 Respiratory therapy	[ ]	[ ]	[ ]	[ ]	[ ]
32 Physical therapy	[ ]	[ ]	[ ]	[ ]	[ ]
33 Social service	[ ]	[ ]	[ ]	[ ]	[ ]
34 Escort service	[ ]	[ ]	[ ]	[ ]	[ ]
35 Chaplaincy	[ ]	[ ]	[ ]	[ ]	[ ]
36 Volunteer	[ ]	[ ]	[ ]	[ ]	[ ]
	1	2	3	4	5

Comments

Your Room:

	Exc.	Good	Fair	Poor
	1	2	3	4
11 Clean	[ ]	[ ]	[ ]	[ ]
12 Quiet	[ ]	[ ]	[ ]	[ ]
13 Comfortable temperature	[ ]	[ ]	[ ]	[ ]
14 Housekeeping service	[ ]	[ ]	[ ]	[ ]

Comments _____

Your Physician(s):

	Exc.	Good	Fair	Poor
	1	2	3	4
15 Concerned	[ ]	[ ]	[ ]	[ ]
16 Courteous	[ ]	[ ]	[ ]	[ ]
17 Clearly explained your medical care and condition	[ ]	[ ]	[ ]	[ ]
18 Posthospital care instructions	[ ]	[ ]	[ ]	[ ]

Comments _____

Your Nursing Care:

	Exc.	Good	Fair	Poor
	1	2	3	4
19 Efficient	[ ]	[ ]	[ ]	[ ]
20 Prompt	[ ]	[ ]	[ ]	[ ]
21 Courteous	[ ]	[ ]	[ ]	[ ]
22 Understanding	[ ]	[ ]	[ ]	[ ]

Comments _____

Your Stay:

	Yes	No		
	1	2		
37 Did you receive patient handbook?	[ ]	[ ]		

	Exc.	Good	Fair	Poor
	1	2	3	4
38 Hospitality extended to you and your visitors	[ ]	[ ]	[ ]	[ ]
39 Professional behavior of hospital personnel	[ ]	[ ]	[ ]	[ ]

Comments _____

Your General Perception:

	Exc.	Good	Fair	Poor
	1	2	3	4
40 Overall impression of hospital and care	[ ]	[ ]	[ ]	[ ]

	Yes	No	
	1	2	
41 If future hospitalization is required, would you select our hospital?	[ ]	[ ]	

Comments _____

Name _____ (Optional)

Address _____ (Optional)

I occupied room # _____ Date of admission _____

Length of stay (check one)

1-2 days [ ] 3-6 days [ ]
7-10 days [ ] 11 or more days [ ]

No. _____

responds to the patients' questions. The 687-bed hospital sees about 130 patients daily in its emergency department. Nurse communicators call more than 100 former patients a day, five days a week. Hospital leaders are convinced that the public relations, patient satisfaction, and quality assurance benefits make the callback system worth the money.

To be sure that postdischarge interviews are effective, you need to:

- *Have a sensitive person do these interviews.* Many hospitals train graduate students or hospital volunteers, other hospitals have nurses make these calls, and still others divide up calls among administrators. Also, market research firms with specially trained interviewers can make these calls, for instance, quarterly.
- *Follow up.* To encourage complaints, you need to have the interviewer promise absolute confidentiality and ask the patient's permission to follow up on the complaint.

Patient Focus Groups

Focus groups, which are richly informative and qualitative methods, are carefully designed and facilitated group discussions intended to assess perceptions held by a customer group and to test responses to new ideas and approaches. As a patient feedback device, focus groups can be used to learn about patients' experience with your organization and their suggestions for improvement.

Linda DeWolf, director of patient and community services at St. Luke's Hospital in Cedar Rapids, Iowa, established an excellent system of patient focus groups run by patient representatives. Other hospitals prefer to use experienced focus-group facilitators or hire them to train in-house people to use state-of-the-art focus group facilitation techniques (Ellen Tobin, "Do-It-Yourself Focus Groups," 10233 Hickory Ridge Road, Suite 202, Columbia, Maryland, 21044, and Jack Fein, the Einstein Consulting Group, York and Tabor Roads, Philadelphia, Pennsylvania 19141).

Figure 7-2 describes St. Luke's focus group program. DeWolf sends the letter in figure 7-3 on hospital stationery to patients who have agreed to participate in the focus groups. For more information, see DeWolf's article "Focus Groups: Assessing Patient Satisfaction and Targeting New Services" in the March-April 1985 issue of *Hospital Topics*, (63[2]:24-26).

Assessing Perceptions of Family Members and Other Visitors

Because visitors and family members are frequently anxious about

Figure 7-2. Description of a Focus-Group Program

**Patient Representative Department
Focus Groups**

Purpose
To offer posthospitalized patients the opportunity to share their perceptions of their hospital experience.

Policies
1. Composition of focus group:
   A. Six to eight patients (from the same patient area and discharged within a two- to six-week time period) plus a support person of the patient's choice, if desired.
   B. A patient representative acting as coordinator and facilitator.
   C. One representative from the particular patient area, if desired.

2. Format:
   A. Patients will be invited to St. Luke's for a light supper or refreshments with group discussion of the hospital experience to follow.

3. Preparation:
   A. Food Service shall be responsible for preparing any meals or refreshments for the group.
   B. Housekeeping shall be responsible for setting up the facility.

4. Follow Up:
   A. The Patient Representative Department shall be responsible for initiating follow up on any voiced concerns.

Procedures
1. Focus group members will be selected from a random sample of former patients (using the criteria established above).

2. Persons shall receive a personal phone call extended by the Patient Representative Department and followed by a letter of invitation.

3. Feedback regarding group discussions shall routinely be provided to administration, quality assurance, and the appropriate patient areas.

4. Routine evaluations of the process shall be conducted by the Patient Representative Department.

Reprinted with permission of St Luke's Hospital, Cedar Rapids, Iowa.

their loved ones, feedback methods should be gentle and should be conducted with extreme tact and discretion. The prospective respondent should clearly understand that participation is entirely optional.

The simple method of *visitor-in-the-hall interviews* can do the job quite well. If conducted properly, these interviews seem more like a chat with a concerned person than an interview. This type of interview can enable you to see your organization from an invaluable perspective. You may just learn something vital about how to make your hospital a better place for visitors and family members, who are

Figure 7-3. Letter Sent to Patients Participating in a Focus Group

Date

Dear _____:

As follow-up to our phone conversation, we are so delighted that you have accepted our invitation to join us here on _____, from 7:00 - 8:30 p.m. for a time of sharing.

We have extended this invitation to only a few persons who were hospitalized during approximately the same time and in the same patient area as you were. We are really looking forward to meeting with you, and a guest of your choice if you'd like, and having an opportunity to discuss your perceptions of your care. Suggestions, comments, and criticisms all will be welcome!

If you should have any further questions about this meeting, please feel free to contact me.

Someone will greet you in the lobby and escort you to the meeting room the evening of the _____.

Sincerely,

Linda DeWolf, Director
Patient and Community Services
369-7710

Reprinted with permission of St Luke's Hospital, Cedar Rapids, Iowa.

too often overlooked as a customer group.

You should begin by politely excusing yourself and then asking individual visitors if they would be willing to share any comments they may have on how to improve your organization. The following is what you might say in such an interview:

Pardon me. I'm _____ from the _____ Department here at the hospital. I'm trying to touch base with visitors to our hospital to see what they think of their experience with us. Would you mind if I ask you a couple of short questions on the way to your car?

- Have you been visiting someone here?
- How are they doing?
- How has your experience with us been?
- How does the patient you've been visiting feel about his or her experience with us?
- Based on your experience here and what the patient you're visiting

may have told you, what could we be doing to improve?

Measuring Physician Perceptions

Physicians, who are a key customer group, make what many people still agree is the lion's share of decisions about which hospitals and ambulatory care services consumers use. At the very least, they influence consumer choice dramatically. Therefore, the answer to the following question is vital: how satisfied are your physicians with the people and services in your organization that influence their ability to serve their patients?

With a systematic evaluation strategy geared to tap physician perceptions, you can:

- Measure the effects of your strategy for service excellence on physicians' perceptions of employee behavior.
- Raise physician awareness of the value your organization places on excellent customer relations.
- Solicit input so you can stay in touch with their views of what makes it easy and hard to practice in your institution.
- Gain information on your strengths and problems so you can modify and focus your ongoing strategy.

Getting information from physicians is not easy, but you can get results if you ask questions and act on what you're hearing. To get information, you may use one or several methods: simple mail surveys, phone interviews, extensive surveys, or focus groups.

Simple Mail Survey

A simple one-page questionnaire (figure 7-4) can help raise physician awareness of your strategy for service excellence, provide you with a rough reading of physicians' perceptions of change, and obtain physician perceptions of problems that need monitoring or solving. Distribute the questionnaire to a sample of physicians before you implement your strategy and at periodic intervals later.

The questionnaire can be mailed with a cover letter on hospital letterhead stationery. Figure 7-5 shows an example of such a cover letter. Remember to include a self-addressed, and preferably stamped, return envelope.

Phone Interviews

Another technique is to telephone a random sample of physicians to

Figure 7-4. Physician Questionnaire on Customer Relations

Physician Survey on HOSPITALity				
	Almost Always	Often	Occasionally	Rarely
1. How often do you think our employees are courteous and helpful to patients?				
2. How often do you think our employees are courteous and helpful to physicians?				
3. What are your patients telling you about the service they receive at our hospital and the courtesy our employees extend to them?				
4. What do you see as the biggest problems our employees have in their interactions with patients?				
5. What do you see as the biggest problems our employees have in their interactions with physicians?				
6. What do you see as the biggest problems our employees have in their interactions with fellow employees?				
7. Any other observations or advice about problems we need to address in our HOSPITALity effort?				
We've provided a return envelope for your convenience. Please return to:				

Reprinted with permission of the Albert Einstein Healthcare Foundation.

find out how they think your employees and your institution are faring in service excellence. You can call before you initiate your customer relations strategy if you do not already have a functioning strategy, and at regular intervals, perhaps quarterly, thereafter.

At the Albert Einstein Medical Center, we called 20 physicians from different departments on a quarterly basis. We stratified our sample of callees so that we could reach high, medium, and low admitters. We asked each callee 5 to 10 minutes' worth of questions about their perceptions of our HOSPITALity program.

In our base-line interview, we told them about our plans to conduct the HOSPITALity effort and asked them to describe from their point of view the strengths and weaknesses in employee behavior to date.

Figure 7-5. Cover Letter to Accompany a Physician Questionnaire

(Cover letter: On Letterhead - Sent with Return Envelope)
TO: (Physician's Name)
FROM:
DATE:
SUBJECT: Your Evaluation of Customer Relations at _____
                                                                                    (Hospital's Name)

As you might have heard, we are launching a comprehensive effort to improve the hospitality extended by our employees to physicians, patients, visitors, and other employees.

To guide our efforts, we are asking a select group of physicians to evaluate the hospitality shown by our employees. You have interacted with many employees, and you have heard patients and family members describe their experience with our personnel.

I'm asking that you complete the short, enclosed questionnaire and return it as soon as possible in the return envelope provided. Your perceptions will help us in our efforts to improve the hospitality we extend to our guests.

Thank you very much for your valuable help.

We also asked them to compare employee behavior in our hospital with that in other hospitals. They were also asked to describe the kinds of comments their patients make about employee behavior and service at our hospital and to include compliments and complaints.

Three months after our initial HOSPITALity workshops, we conducted another round of telephone interviews with physicians. In these interviews, we asked physicians the extent to which they had perceived changes in employee behavior toward their patients, toward one another, toward visitors, and toward the physicians themselves.

Extensive Survey of Physician as Customer

You can also survey physicians in their role as *user* of your organization's services. In their role as user, they deserve and expect excellent service from staff and systems. They call it *ease of practice*. Physicians tend to be more cooperative with staff and more emotionally available to patients if they are not constantly frustrated in their interaction with systems and people. They want what you want: a user-friendly hospital. The survey shown in figure 7-6 was developed at the Albert Einstein Medical Center to get physicians' views of specific services that they rely on to serve their patients. If you can find out what these services are and improve them to make practicing at your facility easier, or user friendly, for the doctor, you have a doctor

Figure 7-6. Extensive Physician Survey

Albert Einstein Medical Center
Northern Division

Physician's Assessment of Northern Division Services

Please indicate your assessment of Northern Division Services by circling the appropriate response. Please use the lines below each section for additional comments.

Rating scale columns (left to right): Excellent / Good / Acceptable / Marginal / Poor / Not applicable / No comment — circled as 5 4 3 2 1 0

Patient Care Services

1. Anesthesiology
   2. availability of personnel — 5 4 3 2 1 0
   3. communication with attending physician — 5 4 3 2 1 0
   4. adequacy of patient preparation — 5 4 3 2 1 0
   5. quality of patient follow-up — 5 4 3 2 1 0

   _____

   _____

6. Operating Room
   7. efficiency of scheduling — 5 4 3 2 1 0
   8. availability of supplies and equipment — 5 4 3 2 1 0
   9. adequacy of patient preparation — 5 4 3 2 1 0
   10. nursing staff follows orders promptly — 5 4 3 2 1 0
   11. nursing staff follows orders correctly — 5 4 3 2 1 0

   _____

12. Intensive Care Unit
   13. quality of intensive care facilities — 5 4 3 2 1 0
   14. adequacy of nursing personnel — 5 4 3 2 1 0
   15. nursing staff follows orders promptly/correctly — 5 4 3 2 1 0
   16. adequacy of house staff coverage — 5 4 3 2 1 0
   17. responsiveness of house staff to attendings' needs — 5 4 3 2 1 0

   _____

18. Recovery Room
   19. efficiency of scheduling — 5 4 3 2 1 0
   20. availability of supplies/equipment — 5 4 3 2 1 0
   21. nursing staff follows orders promptly/correctly — 5 4 3 2 1 0
   22. quality of postoperative care — 5 4 3 2 1 0
   23. quality of documentation of patient information — 5 4 3 2 1 0

   _____

   _____

24. Cardiac Rehabilitation Program
   25. quality of documentation of patient information — 5 4 3 2 1 0
   26. nonphysician staff follows orders promptly/correctly — 5 4 3 2 1 0
   27. communication with referring physicians — 5 4 3 2 1 0
   28. flexibility of scheduling outpatients — 5 4 3 2 1 0
   29. accessibility of facility — 5 4 3 2 1 0
   30. courtesy of nonphysician personnel — 5 4 3 2 1 0

   _____

31. Dialysis
   32. nonphysician staff follows orders promptly/correctly — 5 4 3 2 1 0
   33. communication with referring physicians — 5 4 3 2 1 0
   34. flexibility of scheduling outpatients — 5 4 3 2 1 0
   35. accessibility of facility — 5 4 3 2 1 0
   36. courtesy of nonphysician personnel — 5 4 3 2 1 0

   _____

37. EKG Service (Heart Station)
   38. provide test and results in timely fashion — 5 4 3 2 1 0
   39. variety of procedures/tests available — 5 4 3 2 1 0
   40. ability to discuss interpretation with attending cardiologist — 5 4 3 2 1 0
   41. flexibility of scheduling for outpatients — 5 4 3 2 1 0
   42. responsiveness to needs of attending staff — 5 4 3 2 1 0
   43. courtesy of nonphysician personnel — 5 4 3 2 1 0

   _____

   _____

(continued)

Figure 7-6. *(continued)*

44. EEG Service
45. provide test and results in a timely fashion — 5 4 3 2 1 0
46. variety of procedures/tests available — 5 4 3 2 1 0
47. ability to discuss interpretation with attending neurologist — 5 4 3 2 1 0
48. flexibility of scheduling for outpatients — 5 4 3 2 1 0
49. responsiveness to needs of attending staff — 5 4 3 2 1 0
50. courtesy of nonphysician personnel — 5 4 3 2 1 0

———————————————

51. Emergency Unit
52. promptness of response to patients' needs — 5 4 3 2 1 0
53. observation of patients during entire E.R. stay — 5 4 3 2 1 0
54. adequacy of communication with waiting family and friends — 5 4 3 2 1 0
55. provide test and results of x-ray and lab studies in a timely fashion — 5 4 3 2 1 0
56. responsive to needs of attending staff — 5 4 3 2 1 0
57. courtesy of nonphysician personnel — 5 4 3 2 1 0

———————————————

58. Laboratory
59. accuracy of laboratory studies — 5 4 3 2 1 0
60. provide test and results in a timely fashion — 5 4 3 2 1 0
61. variety of tests/procedures available — 5 4 3 2 1 0
62. responsiveness to new technologies — 5 4 3 2 1 0
63. ability to discuss interpretation with responsible lab personnel — 5 4 3 2 1 0
64. courtesy of nonphysician personnel — 5 4 3 2 1 0

———————————————

65. Preadmission Testing
66. follow orders correctly — 5 4 3 2 1 0
67. provide test and results in a timely fashion — 5 4 3 2 1 0

68. courtesy of personnel — 5 4 3 2 1 0
69. hours of operation — 5 4 3 2 1 0

———————————————

70. Nursing Staff (refers to nurses only)
71. professional skill of personnel — 5 4 3 2 1 0
72. efficiency/courtesy of personnel — 5 4 3 2 1 0
73. follow orders promptly/correctly — 5 4 3 2 1 0
74. alertness to complications — 5 4 3 2 1 0
75. adequacy of communication with attending physicians — 5 4 3 2 1 0
76. quality of reporting on patient chart — 5 4 3 2 1 0

———————————————

77. Pharmacy
78. adequacy of formulary — 5 4 3 2 1 0
79. medication dispensed accurately from pharmacy — 5 4 3 2 1 0
80. attention to patient sensitivity or other contraindications — 5 4 3 2 1 0
81. adequacy of communication with attending physician — 5 4 3 2 1 0
82. knowledgability about potential drug hazards or shortages — 5 4 3 2 1 0

———————————————

83. Radiology
84. provide test and results in a timely fashion — 5 4 3 2 1 0
85. variety of procedures/tests available — 5 4 3 2 1 0
86. ability to discuss interpretation with attending radiologist — 5 4 3 2 1 0
87. flexibility of scheduling for outpatients — 5 4 3 2 1 0
88. responsiveness to new technologies — 5 4 3 2 1 0
89. promptness of performing patient x-ray at scheduled time — 5 4 3 2 1 0
90. responsiveness to needs of attending staff — 5 4 3 2 1 0

———————————————

(continued)

Figure 7-6. *(continued)*

Support Services

We are interested in receiving your comments about nonclinical as well as clinical hospital services with respect to the support services listed below. Please let us know your impressions about personnel courtesy, competence, efficiency, and responsiveness of the following:

(Use the lines below each department for additional comments.)
(Please use back of sheet for additional comments.)

	No comment / Not applicable / Poor / Marginal / Acceptable / Good / Excellent
91 Admissions	5 4 3 2 1 0
92. Business Office/Cashier	5 4 3 2 1 0
93. Cafeteria	5 4 3 2 1 0
94 Escort Service	5 4 3 2 1 0
95 Info/Mail	5 4 3 2 1 0
96 Medical Library	5 4 3 2 1 0
97 Medical Records	5 4 3 2 1 0

Reprinted with permission of Albert Einstein Medical Center, Northern Division.

more likely to direct patients to your institution and more appreciative of your people.

Physician Focus Groups

As with patient focus groups, physician focus groups can yield rich, qualitative results. If you want to know how user friendly your organization really is, just ask physicians these questions:

- What about a hospital encourages you to admit patients?
- What discourages you from admitting patients?
- What encourages you about the way our hospital operates?
- What discourages you about the way our hospital operates?

A focus group works best with targeted, or homogenous, groups. For example, a group can be composed of physicians who are low admitters or medium admitters or high admitters or nonadmitters or former admitters or residents, but not combinations of these physicians.

Ideally, an outside, disinterested party with focus-group facilitation skills should conduct the group. Physicians may be more comfortable when the person conducting the group has no vested interest in the outcome and so will maintain confidentiality. Usually the session is taped, or someone takes extensive notes for later analysis. Be sure that the participants understand beforehand that the proceedings is being taped or that notes are being taken.

Sometimes hospitals hire a focus-group professional to conduct two or three focus groups and tape the sessions. Then they use the focus-group tapes to train a local, less expensive facilitator to conduct groups on a regular basis. If you don't want to use outsiders, choose skillful, open-minded, and trusted staff members.

Another way to work with a physician focus group is to use the Customer Service Matrix (figure 7-7). Explain the Customer Service Matrix and ask physicians to point out strengths and weaknesses in selected boxes.

Figure 7-7. Customer Service Matrix

| Key Components | Customer Groups | | | | |
	Patients	Visitors	Physicians	Employees	Third-Party Payers
Technical competence					
Environment					
People skills					
Systems					
Amenities					

Assessing Employee Perceptions and Satisfaction

The group with the most firsthand experience with your organization's people, systems, customers, and outcomes is your employees. You dare not overlook the perceptions and experiences of this group because they are a top-notch source of information and because not to ask their views devalues employees and dims their commitment and sense of ownership in your organization. Employees are the key to service excellence and, consequently, to the organization's image in the professional and patient community; in other words, employees are the key to your organization's success.

By focusing evaluation techniques on employees as care givers and as customers, you can:

- Identify the effects of your strategy for service excellence on employee behavior, morale, and pride in the organization.
- Target strengths and problems that help focus your future strategies.
- Welcome employee participation in identifying strengths and achievements that deserve acknowledgment as well as problems that cry for attention.
- Focus on ways to help employees feel better served and more satisfied as recipients of service by coworkers.
- Identify ways your organization can help your employees feel recognized, appreciated, and cared for.

You can use a variety of methods, singly or in combination, to measure employee perceptions and satisfaction:

- *Behavior self-report.* If your strategy for service excellence promotes specific behavior, you can ask employees how often they and their coworkers exhibit these specific behaviors. Administer such a survey before the strategy is instituted and at periodic intervals later. At Albert Einstein Medical Center, we built into our initial three-hour HOSPITALity workshop a "Taking Stock" survey to tap employee perceptions of employee behavior (figure 7-8). The survey asks employees to comment on the frequency of each of our HOSPITALity "House Rule" behaviors on the part of coworkers and themselves.
- *Workshop evaluation.* Every customer relations workshop you sponsor is an opportunity to collect valuable employee perceptions. Incorporate questions on pride, loyalty, and the like.
- *Post-only survey.* If you already have an explicit strategy for service excellence, you can't obtain base-line information from your

Figure 7-8. Part of the "Taking Stock" Survey Form

Taking Stock: Your Impressions of HOSPITALity

I. What's your sense of how often *employees* show the following behaviors?

		Hardly Ever	A Little	A Lot	Almost Always	Not in a Position Do This
A	Employees smile at patients, visitors, and one another.					
B	Employees make eye contact with patients, visitors, and one another.					
C	Employees introduce themselves to patients.					
D	Employees call people by name.					
E	Employees help people who look confused.					

I. What's your sense of how often *you* show the following behaviors?

		Hardly Ever	A Little	A Lot	Almost Always	Not in a Position Do This
A	I smile at patients, visitors, and coworkers.					
B	I make eye contact with patients, visitors, and coworkers.					
C	I introduce myself to patients.					
D	I call people by name.					
E	I help people who look confused.					

Reprinted with permission of the Albert Einstein Healthcare Foundation.

employees. However, you can still learn from them in a post-only (figure 7-9) and then periodic survey. Ask straightforward perception questions to all or a sample of employees at periodic intervals after you institute your strategy. Although such research isn't fancy, it does give you a reading on whether employees think your strategy is beneficial.

- *Interdepartmental service evaluation.* Employees are, or need to be, customers to one another. An enlightened customer relations strategy raises employee awareness and builds skills that should translate into better service extended by one department to another, one employee to another.

  "Get off my back. Can't you see I'm on break?" said one employee to another who needed supplies from the supply room during a code blue. Not only is that behavior antipatient; it's also unacceptable teamwork between employees. Employees must begin to see one another as customers who merit responsive, attentive help and concern.

  Consider a survey like the one in figure 7-10 to assess interdepartmental perceptions of perhaps 10 departments at a time. Within a month, all departments should be subjected to peer evaluation.

- *Focus groups.* Focus groups tend to win the evaluation-method popularity contest. They produce substantive, in-depth information and gather this information in a participatory style that promotes face-to-face communication. Such face-to-face communication reflects the philosophy and soul of service excellence. Ask people to talk about what they think and feel, and they'll do so frankly and constructively.

  A focus group should have anywhere from 12 to 40 participants. Begin by explaining your intention to make organizational improvements with their help. Post and explain the Customer Service Matrix (figure 7-7). Ask people to form groups of three or four persons and to identify specific strengths and weaknesses in what they consider to be the most important boxes of the matrix. Reconvene the entire group and invite a sharing of each group's results. Then, and this step is the key, tell people what will be done to improve the problems that the group thinks are important.

- *Attitude survey.* Attitude surveys are popular evaluation devices. Although attitude is nebulous and not necessarily correlated with behavior, attitude surveys can still be useful. Typically, organizations hire outside research firms to conduct them. A word of warning: don't conduct an attitude survey unless you're clear about your purpose and your strategy for following up on results. You'll take "10 steps backward" if you give people a chance to let off steam and then do nothing about the steam. Even the employees who

Figure 7-9. Post-Only Survey

HOSPITALity: Questionnaire to Employees

You are in a select group of people. We are surveying a sample of 200 employees, and you have been selected to be a part of a survey of our HOSPITALity effort. As you know, we have been working to improve the HOSPITALity we extend to guests of our hospital: We'd like to know if you've seen any change in HOSPITALity over the last three months. Please fill this out and return it to _____ in the enclosed envelope.

Changes	Worse	Same as Before	A Little Better	A Lot Better
From employees How much change have you seen in employee hospitality toward patients?				
How much change have you seen in employee hospitality toward visitors?				
How much change have you seen in employee hospitality toward doctors?				
How much change have you seen in employee hospitality toward fellow employees?				
From doctors How much change have you seen in doctors' hospitality toward patients?				
How much change have you seen in doctors' hospitality toward visitors?				
How much change have you seen in doctors' hospitality toward employees?				
From yourself How much change have you seen in your hospitality toward patients?				
How much change have you seen in your hospitality toward visitors?				
How much change have you seen in your hospitality toward doctors?				
How much change have you seen in your hospitality toward fellow employees?				

4. What are the biggest changes you've seen since the HOSPITALity effort began?
_____
_____

(continued)

Figure 7-9. *(continued)*

Suggestion Boxes

5. Have you seen the HOSPITALity suggestion boxes?   Yes ____   No ____
6. Have you used the boxes to make your ideas or
   feelings known?   Yes ____   No ____

Comments: _____

_____

HOSPITALity News

7. Have you seen the HOSPITALity newsletter?   Yes ____   No ____
8. Did you find the newsletter interesting?   Yes ____   No ____

Comments: _____

_____

HOSPITALity Posters

9. Have you seen the HOSPITALity posters?   Yes ____   No ____
10 Do you like them?   Yes ____   No ____

Comments: _____

_____

Other Ideas

11. What ideas do you have for how we can continue to improve our HOSPITALity?

Comments: _____

_____

Reprinted with permission of the Albert Einstein Healthcare Foundation

Figure 7-10.   Survey to Assess Interdepartmental Perceptions

---

Department Name: _____

very low					**very high**
Staff courtesy/helpfulness:					
1	2	3	4	5	6
Efficiency of operations:					
1	2	3	4	5	6
Accuracy of tasks performed:					
1	2	3	4	5	6
Comments and suggestions:					

Reprinted with permission of the Albert Einstein Healthcare Foundation adopt a wait-and-see attitude gradually come to feel patronized and resentful.

- *Exit interviews.* When employees resign, your personnel people should arrange for an exit interview. These interviews help you gain valuable information about your organization, certain departments, and quality-of-work-life issues that affect your organization's ability to achieve service excellence. Also, if you consider the employee a customer, exit interviews can make an employee's departure more amicable. After all, a former employee spreads the word about your organization and is therefore an ambassador of goodwill or bad will. Former employees are more likely to speak well of your organization if you do all you can to make their departure pleasant and if you recognize and respect them as intelligent, astute individuals.

Assessing the Satisfaction of Third-party Payers

Unions, employers, insurance companies, HMOs, and PPOs all want to do business with a high-quality, cost-effective, user-friendly health care provider who is responsive to their requests for service, access, and information. Focus groups can serve to identify the critical issues that affect the satisfaction of these third-party payers. You can then follow up with periodic, perhaps annual or semiannual, telephone or mail surveys to keep you informed about the important perceptions and needs of third-party payers.

In your focus groups or surveys, you can ask the following questions:

- What do you look for in a hospital? What factors need to exist to attract you to do business with one hospital versus another?
- How do you view this hospital as a health care provider? What makes this hospital attractive or unattractive to you?
- What are your frustrations when dealing with this hospital?
- What do your members or constituents or subscribers or employees say about this hospital?
- How could this hospital improve its effectiveness in your eyes and, consequently, its relationship with you?

Scuttlebutt Evaluation and Other Valuable Evaluation Methods

Apart from the methods described earlier in this chapter that tap each major customer group, other methods, for instance, suggestion boxes, outsider's perspectives, and scuttlebutt, can provide valuable information.

Put a *suggestion box* in a prominent place on each patient floor and major public area and encourage people to use it. To make it convenient, attach a pad of paper with a headline like the following: "Help Us Make Things Better." Suggestion boxes are a great way to get invaluable feedback on how you're doing and what you could be doing even better.

Try an *outsider's perspective*. Citizens' groups, volunteers, peers from a sister organization, and people from businesses with a strong tradition of service can provide you with information from a unique perspective. Ask them to visit and observe and to be your consultants on ways to advance toward service excellence. Consider using the expertise of hotel managers by asking them to tour your facility and answer the question "If this were your hotel, what changes would you make?" You can also learn by visiting their hotels and examining their customer relations policies. Talk to other customer-oriented business people, including restaurant managers, retailers, and airline personnel. Consulting firms can also provide an experienced, outsider's eye view of your organization.

Don't discount *scuttlebutt* as an evaluation technique. Collect anecdotes, complimentary letters, and complaints from every source in order to evaluate your strategy for service excellence. Scrutinize the comments, complaints, and suggestions to learn how people feel about the services rendered to them by your organization.

In addition to these methods, you can expect to evaluate your strategy for service excellence by examining the feelings of people who have experienced major components of your strategy. Certain behavior patterns may dramatically and obviously change. For instance, at Albert Einstein Medical Center, we couldn't help but notice that four or five people approached a visitor who appeared lost or disoriented to see if they could be of help. This reaction was an obvious result of our initial wave of workshops. You and your colleagues experience your environment on a day-to-day basis and witness changes that happen as a result of your strategy for service excellence. Don't discount these observations. They are reality, and they are informative.

☐ Final Suggestions

Consider these suggestions when evaluating your systems for input and evaluation:

- *Be wary of unfair criteria.* Don't use unfair criteria to evaluate your strategy for service excellence. Ask yourself if the proposed indicator is influenced by any factors that may overwhelm the effects of even a strong strategy for service excellence. For example, every hospital wants to increase patient volume or admissions. However, admissions and patient volume should not be used to evaluate the results of your strategy because too many variables affect it. You may have declining hospital admissions after implementing your strategy for service excellence. Can you say with certainty that your strategy caused the decline? Without your strategy, admissions may have declined even faster. Perhaps your strategy helped to stem the tide.

  Although market share is a better indicator than admissions or patient volume, it too is influenced by so many other strategies and forces. For this reason, focus your evaluation on *perceptions* of staff behavior and customer satisfaction with service. *Focus your evaluation on what your strategy can affect directly.* To take liberties with an old Irish prayer, "Give me the energy to control what I can, the courage to let go of what I can't, and the wisdom to know the difference."

- *Press for a substantive, ongoing customer survey.* Administrators who think they know what customers think without asking them are mistaken. With a systematic survey, administrators and others will unfailingly learn a lot and have the credibility of actual data to support their efforts to address problems.

- *Worry if you can't get support for evaluation.* Ongoing evaluation or input from your customers is your lifeline. If your administrative team won't dedicate resources to evaluation, find a quiet room and meditate seriously on top management's commitment to service excellence. If top managers won't pay for good evaluation, they are only paying lip service to service excellence.

- *Beware of dogged insistence on research purity.* If you read textbooks about research, you see admonitions about "dirtying" the data by impure methods. Is it really sensible to delegate staying close to your customers to pure researchers, to outsiders with detachment and objectivity? Consider instead the maverick view that *evaluation and input-gathering techniques should be obtrusive interventions that reinforce your employees' and physicians' service orientation and that make them self-conscious about how they're treating customers.* Methods for tapping patient and visitor perceptions should also be obtrusive to show that your organization cares and wants to excel in meeting their needs. You may need to let go of academic notions of research in order to build a comprehensive, educational evaluation strategy that keeps your organization on the road toward service excellence.

- *Your strategy doesn't have to be a Cadillac to keep you rolling forward.* Some people give themselves headaches because of all the things they know they should do in the way of evaluating but that they can't see their way clear to doing all at once. Don't worry about what you can't do. Be concerned about what you can do. *Start somewhere:* Something is better than nothing. Start with a rough draft of an evaluation strategy and make improvements as you use it.

Systems for input and evaluation replace mind reading with fact. Knowing the perceptions and level of satisfaction of every customer group—patients, family and other visitors, physicians, employees, and third-party payers—provides invaluable information that you can use to guide your strategy for service excellence and lend it the credibility of accountability for results.

Problem Solving and Complaint Management

Problems and complaints are inevitable. If you ask patients, visitors, doctors, and employees to voice them, or even if you don't, problems of every shape and consequence rear their agonizing heads. The better your systems of input gathering and evaluation, the more you'll learn about problems that interfere with your customers' satisfaction.

Take the test in figure 8-1 to get an idea of how your hospital stacks up on problem solving and complaint management. The more "yes" answers, the better. "No" answers point to gaps in your systems for problem solving and complaint management.

This chapter summarizes the whys and wherefores of strong problem-solving and complaint-management systems. It examines the roles of management and employees, a team approach, and problem-solving techniques. It then focuses on the importance of effective complaint management. Then because health care organizations are highly specialized and complex and as a result may have overwhelming systems problems, the chapter looks at these systems problems in particular and their powerful impact on service excellence.

□ Problem Solving and Service Excellence

The obvious fact is that problems interfere with customer satisfaction, and so they must be solved or you are going to have dissatisfied customers. Problems must also be taken seriously because they have

Figure 8-1. Self-Test: How Effective Are Your Problem-Solving and Complaint-Management Systems?

Problem-Solving and Complaint-Management Systems. Circle the appropriate answer. The more "yes" answers, the better. "No" answers indicate areas that need improvement.

1. Generally, your staff members welcome and invite customer complaints because complaints give them a chance to show their concern and responsiveness. Yes No

2. Generally, your staff members are apologetic and concerned when patients are not satisfied; staff members bend over backward to resolve complaints. Yes No

3. When patients have a complaint or concern, they know whom to call. Yes No

4. You have a clear system for handling patient complaints and needs. Yes No

5. You have a system for communicating back to patients any actions taken as a result of their complaints or requests. Yes No

6. When employees have complaints or suggestions, they know specific channels for expressing them. Yes No

7. Your administration and middle managers generally respond to employee complaints and concerns, even if they don't fix them. Yes No

8. Your administration is generally perceived as open to employee complaints and suggestions. Yes No

9. Information on patient perceptions and problems is channeled to the right people for consideration, problem solving, and action. Yes No

10. Physician complaints and suggestions are fed into a clear process for consideration, problem solving, and action. Yes No

11. Employee complaints and suggestions are channeled to the right people for consideration, problem solving, and action. Yes No

12. Your employees believe in speaking up because they know that someone is listening. Yes No

13. In your organization, managers at every level are actively responsible for taking action on problems that interfere with customers' satisfaction. Yes No

Figure 8-1. *(continued)*

14. In your organization, employees closest to the job are actively involved in solving problems that relate to their jobs.	Yes No
15. You have a culture in which employee participation in problem solving is a usual practice.	Yes No
16. Your employees have confidence that your administrators won't ignore important problems brought to their attention; they may not solve them, but they won't ignore them.	Yes No
17. You have patient representatives, advocates, or others whose job is to intervene in and facilitate problem solving.	Yes No
Total:	___ ___

to do with employee morale and pride. Says Gail Scott of the Einstein Consulting Group: "Underneath it all, employees want to do a great job. And they want to be proud of their organization. No one is happy about the customers who choose to go elsewhere because of dissatisfaction. No one likes watching business walk away toward the hospital down the street. And no one likes to feel defeated by the mountain of problems their organization perpetuates day after day."

In a telephone conversation in October 1987, Columbia University professor James Kuhn points out one reason for growing discontent among American workers: "Most people like to think that they are doing something important and valuable and making a contribution. To be forced by management to ignore that value takes away from the enjoyment of the job. In many cases, you find that workers feel strongly about product quality, but they just can't do anything about it."

This worker attitude is probably even more important in health care, where many, and probably most, employees chose the field because they want to help people. Then they find themselves having to implement processes and procedures that are not helpful to customers; and when they complain, they can't seem to jiggle the system. They become disaffected and angry. Here they are, thinking about what's best for the customer, and top management is glued tenaciously to the dime and is unwilling to tackle problems or make changes that make things better for everyone. Then what happens? Employee commitment to service excellence and their willingness to work hard for the organization diminishes.

How open are you to hearing about problems? Three patterns are indications of closed-mindedness in hospitals:

- Comfort with the status quo
- Employee as meddler
- The immune response

Consider first the idea of *being comfortable with the status quo.* How often have you sensed the attitude that "if it's not broken, don't fix it," or "if it's just a bit broken, wait till it falls apart completely, and maybe that will happen after I'm long gone." These attitudes are perhaps all too common among management. Why seek out improvements? After all, even little changes take time, need approval, and require alterations in how departments function. Change making takes time away from daily operations, and time is so scarce. No wonder managers take the easy way out unless the incentive or threat is compelling.

Now consider the idea of *employee as meddler.* In any organization, some employees are always trying to make things better. However, some soon learn that they're considered meddlesome if they criticize the way things are or suggest improvements. If you view such employees as whistle-blowers, you frustrate the natural and valuable instinct to build a better mousetrap. Employees get the message: "Even if management says they're open to your ideas, keep your mouth shut."

What about the *immune response.* Problems aren't noticed because employees are so used to them. They've adapted to the policies and practices even if these policies and practices make no sense anymore and fail to serve the customer.

In health care, you have to change all these attitudes and right away. You have to ask:

- Why are you doing this?
- Must you do it this way?
- Can you find a better way to do it?

Once you decide to tackle problems, you can solve them by using standard problem-solving processes.

- Describe the symptoms.
- Get the facts.
- Define the problem.
- Develop alternatives.
- Select the best, although maybe imperfect, alternative.
- Implement it.

The process may seem simple, but using it effectively is admittedly not easy. Institutional language has to change to encourage employees to lower their defensiveness and to feel free to experiment. Problems need to be expressed as opportunities to improve customer satisfaction, and not as hassles that people have created through their own negligence, oversight, and incompetence.

Management must make eminently clear that service excellence is everybody's business and that change on everyone's part is expected. Top management should hold meetings in which they ask middle managers not how things are going, but what changes are being made to improve customer satisfaction.

Management must then recognize and reward employees who develop new methods and then invest time and effort into future-oriented activity. Management needs to create a supportive culture for innovation by middle management and by the entire work force. In *Creating Excellence* (New York City: New American Library, 1985), Craig Hickman and Michael Silva say that creating excellence requires:

- Being willing to drop an approach that isn't working
- Finding ways to force yourself out of habitual methods of thinking or analyzing
- Relentlessly pursuing difficult problems over long periods of time without feeling frustrated or giving up when solutions are not immediately apparent

Once you as executives and managers are aware that a problem exists, what do you do about it? Do you see yourself in the following list? Do you do any of the following?

- Deny it? "I don't see it!"
- Defend yourself? "If you think we don't have reasons for things as they are, you're wrong!"
- Appease? "Thank you, all of you dedicated, concerned people; don't worry, we'll consider it."
- Discount it? "If you think that's a problem, you should see this other mess!"
- Pretend it didn't happen? "What problem? I don't see any big problem here."
- Pawn it off on someone else? "That's not my job."
- Trigger guilt? "Do you honestly believe we did that on purpose? Now, really!"
- Delegate it to someone who may let it drop? "Don't worry, dears. It's in good hands."

- Make promises that you don't mean? "You'll see big things happening to prevent this from ever happening again! Soon!"

What you choose to do with the input, survey results, complaints, and suggestions from every customer group makes the difference between a responsive organization and a stagnant, defensive, and self-satisfied one that, in the face of problems and complaints, erodes customer and employee confidence. According to Morgan McCall, Jr., director of research for the Center of Creative Leadership in Greensboro, North Carolina, the number of mistakes is not what distinguishes Fortune 500 managers from managers who are less successful. The real difference is *their ability to handle mistakes.* Top executives accept responsibility for errors, inform the people affected, and try immediately to correct them. These executives learn from their mistakes. They don't dwell on them, and they continue to take risks and make changes.

Top Management's Role

Top management has four roles in problem solving. It must:

- Install the systems for problem solving.
- Create an organizational culture that supports the effective use of these systems.
- Monitor the results along the way.
- Hold people accountable. Hire people who are creative, nondefensive problem solvers. Reward people who are effective in solving problems and resolving complaints. When necessary, get rid of the people who just don't cut it.

The ultimate responsibility for problem solving is top management's, whether they want it or not. Instead of pointing the finger at middle managers who allow problems to go on year after year, top managers need to either get those middle managers functioning as active, responsible problem-solvers, or they need to get new middle managers. If middle managers are ineffective in actively minimizing problems and solving those they couldn't prevent, even when these problems cut across department lines, then top management has not clarified that problem solving and complaint management are key aspects of the middle manager's job or has tolerated people in middle-management jobs who shouldn't be there. The buck for permitting problems to go on and on to the detriment of the organization and its customers stops with top management.

Top management must somehow actively participate in the chain of events needed to institutionalize, through hands-on leadership, an atmosphere of aggressive problem solving and complaint resolution. Top management specifically needs to:

- Earmark problems that must be solved if the organization is to achieve its goals.
- Identify and assign clear responsibility, perhaps in teams, to tackle each problem, no matter how complex, and provide resources as needed.
- Institute a reporting system so that progress can be tracked and the problem does not fall through any cracks.
- Institute a system for evaluating managers that includes as a critical criterion their performance on problem solving.
- Devote resources to building a team of patient representatives who can find the right people when problems arise and expedite problem solving across departmental lines.
- Take full responsibility for creating a climate for serious problem solving and innovation in order to tackle problems relating to service excellence creatively and with deliberate speed.

Employee Participation

How many outside consultants have been brought in to hospitals to debug departmental procedures that the employees in that department could have streamlined themselves? How many solutions have been foisted on people who do the job by people who don't only to find that in real life, their out-of-touch solutions could not possibly work? The result is employees who feel devalued and discounted when they want to feel appreciated and respected for all they know and for all they could do to improve the organization.

Consider the wisdom of Akio Morita, chairperson of the SONY Corporation, as expressed in *Made in Japan* (New York City: E. P. Dutton, 1986):

> A company will get nowhere if all the thinking is left to management. Everybody in the company must contribute. That means letting low level employees do more than just manual labor. At SONY, we insist that all of our employees contribute their *minds*.

The Team Approach

In the 1970s, everyone talked about participative management.

Everyone from the part-timer to the president was going to get together in work teams and run a profitable, successful, happy family-type corporation. Management asked employees how they could improve their output and then promised to help them do it.

As reported in the July 21, 1986, issue of *Fortune*, a study of 101 industrial companies found participative management to be highly successful at *certain* levels, but its good effects just didn't last. Plans were formed, and they worked in the boiler room. Work teams on the shop floor kept a lot of people happy. Where it all bogged down was in the middle; participation and involvement just couldn't penetrate the middle-management network.

Participation does not sit well with middle management, where traditionalism is usually the most firmly placed. When middle managers see their departments producing satisfactory results, they are reluctant to change their ways because not taking risks is easier and much safer. Middle management seems to fear an immediate undermining of their authority, and authority is seen as an important part of status. As one manager put it succinctly, "If you take my authority away from me, you leave me with a lot of headaches and a salary that's hardly worth having."

Because management teams involve the workers in more decision making and problem solving, workers also become privy to more inside information. Because they know more about what's going on, they may subject the middle manager to pressure from below in addition to the pressure from above. Information is power, and so middle management frequently sees giving away too much information as a weakening of their power.

For the sake of service excellence and its prerequisite—employee morale—you need to take another crack at participatory management. When you enlist employee support for service excellence, employees then understandably expect to be included or at least consulted in decision making about ways to increase customer satisfaction. In the process, middle managers need to stop thinking "if you want this job to get done, you'll have to do it my way" and start thinking "together we can iron out these problems and get these plans under way."

Problem-Solving Systems

A culture that supports problem solving isn't enough. Formal systems are needed so that problems don't fall through cracks. For example, what happens when your patient representatives track complaints and identify recurrent problems? If you form periodic employee focus groups (and let's hope you do) to solicit their views of the service strengths and weaknesses of your organization in your efforts to satisfy patients and if these focus groups generate lists of problems, big and small, complex and seemingly trivial, what do you do with the lists? Listening to the patient representatives and to the focus-group participants isn't enough. You need to take the results and feed them through a process. If you don't, you let valuable information evaporate. You also generate deep resentment among employees and patients who have been led to expect responsiveness.

All hospitals, with the help of their patient representatives, should have ongoing systems for trying to solve the problems of patients and visitors. If your hospital already has such systems, great; if not, consider setting up a system as soon as possible. However, don't forget to include in your system service problems identified by employees.

Here's an example of an explicit system for sorting out problems identified by patient representatives or focus groups and for clearly deciding into which basket each problem goes so that it does not get lost and so that your employees know that the problem was heard and given genuine attention:

- Before the focus group, arrange to tape the meeting or assign someone to take notes so that data are not lost.
- Afterward, glean information from the tapes or notes. First, list each problem cited by category (patient concerns, physician concerns, systems problems, staff concerns). Then, next to each problem, tally the number of times this problem was mentioned or reinforced. With the focus group leader present, code each item also by the *intensity* of the feelings surrounding the item.
- Summarize the results in the form of a report that lists each problem with the frequency and intensity of feelings surrounding it.
- Convene a complaint clearinghouse. Set up a committee of employees, including managers and nonmanagers, to function as a complaint clearinghouse. Have this committee discuss the problems cited in the report and then develop an "if we had our druthers" letter or presentation to the executive team that outlines which set of problems they believe should best be tackled early on.
- The executive team reviews this letter or presentation and the backup data, discusses them, and decides what to do about the problems raised. Specifically, they clearly sort the problems into two groups:
  —Problems the organization is already acting on: These problems include those already solved or about to be solved and those in the process of being tackled.
  —Problems the organization hasn't done anything about yet.

These problems include those to be acted on immediately; those to be investigated further before options can be evaluated; those to be tabled for now either because no solution currently can be found that doesn't create more problems or because the organization can't afford the solution that makes sense; and those to be solved with the help of employee participation or problem-solving teams.

Employees need to be informed of top management's actions relating to each of these various kinds of problems. Top management needs to explain, for example, what solutions are being considered, how a solution is to be implemented, what progress is being made toward finding a solution, or why possible solutions can't effectively be implemented.

This system may not necessarily be the right one for you. The point is that you need *formal systems* for reviewing problems and complaints raised through your various input-gathering vehicles and deciding what you're going to do about them.

Methods for Problem Solving

Consider using such problem-solving methods as quality circles, work teams, ad hoc problem-solving groups, idea contests, and suggestion boxes. Employ within these various structures such analytical and creative techniques as nominal group technique, force-field analysis, brainstorming, value analysis, rank ordering, synectics using metaphoric thinking, pareto analysis, cause and effect analysis, and the like. The following are a few references that provide information on these and other problem-solving techniques:

- *High Involvement Management,* by Edward Lawler (San Francisco, CA: Jossey-Bass, Inc., 1986)
- *Techniques of Structured Problem-Solving,* by Arthur Van Gundy, Jr. (New York City: Van Nostrand Reinhold, 1981)
- *Putting Quality Circles to Work,* by Ralph Barra (New York City: McGraw-Hill Book Co., 1983)

Books, curricula, consultants, and other resources for problem solving abound. The problem is not a shortage of problem-solving resources. The problem is getting management to decide to engage in aggressive problem solving, to make the decision to hunt for problems though most hit you in the face), chase solutions, try them, fix them, and make conditions better. *The problem is to get management to make problem solving a mode of daily operation.*

☐ Complaint Management

As hard as you try to eliminate problems, you will, of course, hear multitudes of complaints from your customers. Complaints are part of any business in which the public interacts with complex systems, and no system is more complex than health care, where care givers, who are only human, work in stressful, emotionally charged situations.

Ironically, whether your organization causes complaints or not is not the main problem. The problem is how customers *perceive your response* once they complain. This perception has a powerful effect on their overall perception of you and your services and on their willingness to choose your hospital for health care the next time. Complainers are more likely than noncomplainers to do business with the organization that upset them even if the problem isn't resolved. Thus, staff, and not only patient representatives, should *always* be available to at least hear complaints. Furthermore, of those who do complain, between 54 percent and 70 percent do business again with the organization if their complaint is resolved, and this figure climbs to be a staggering 95 percent if the customer believes that the complaint was resolved quickly.

According to Gail Scott, director of guest relations services for the Einstein Consulting Group, hospitals are increasingly beginning to scrutinize how customer complaints are handled within their walls. Some hospitals hire specific staff members, such as patient representatives, guest relations directors, and concierges, to handle complaints, and such actions are fine as long as these staff aren't the *only* people expected to do so. Other hospitals are working with middle managers to help every one of them be problem solvers for customers, and this strategy is also good as long as it doesn't stop there. Gail Scott insists that "managers should be concerned and responsible for service excellence, but these persons should not be the only ones concerned. Employees too need to recognize their role as problem solvers. If managers intervene in a problem between employee and customer, the employee and customer are kept at arm's length, and employees may not develop the skills they need to handle tough issues. As a result, they feel less committed, less proud of their own abilities, and less invested in the outcomes of their actions because someone is there to pick up the pieces. Also, managers are not necessarily there when a problem arises. Even if they were, they can't spend all their time putting out fires. They should really be devoting their time to making improvements that would prevent future complaints.

Some organizations are training every employee in their organization to cope effectively with complaints, because they never know when, where, or to whom complaints will be voiced. They realize that "customers are always right even when they're wrong." These organizations understand that complaint management is at least a three-legged stool that also requires administrative support in order to stay upright:

- One leg is managers and supervisors at all levels who must at times get involved in complaint management.
- The second leg is all employees, because every employee should be able to hear complaints nondefensively and with understanding and then either take care of the complaint or refer it to someone who can.
- The third leg, and the one without which the stool topples, is a squad of people dedicated to complaint handling, tracking, and follow-up. These people are the patient representatives or patient advocates. They move the system on the customer's behalf and also serve as catalysts in solving problems after they've occurred.

Every employee should invite complaints and should see them as opportunities, as a second chance to satisfy what would have otherwise been a dissatisfied customer. They should not view complaints as "a bother and a hassle."

Managers and supervisors are charged with reversing this negative employee attitude wherever it exists. Managers and supervisors have to not only become involved in complaint management themselves, but they also need to train their subordinates to handle complaints effectively and to see complaint management as a critical element of their jobs. To effectively equip their people to handle complaints, managers and supervisors need to watch out for the "it's-easier-to-do-it-myself" pattern that works against their employees recognizing problems and taking the initiative to solve them. Some managers are afraid to let others handle complaints or don't trust their people to handle complaints because of past experience. Still others would probably like their people to handle complaints, but they don't know how to teach them to do so.

Managers can foster the atmosphere for effective complaint management by taking the following steps:

- Create a low-threat learning environment for your people.
- Let your employees see you solve a sticky customer service issue. Then review the steps and discuss the techniques you used.
- Develop a repertoire of typical complaints your department hears.

Use these case studies in teaching new employees about complaint management and reviewing skill refinements with employees who have been on the job for a while. Do role plays until people are comfortable handling complaints in a welcoming, nondefensive manner.

- After incidents in which employees have not solved a guest problem effectively, go back over the steps and ask open-ended questions to help the employee see better alternatives.
- Create a rotating "supervisor on call" so that people, not necessarily supervisors, practice helping one another resolve complaints and problems.
- Recognize employee efforts. They may feel awkward as they build their muscles for handling complaints.

As managers work through this learning process with their employees, they need to believe that:

- There's more than one right answer.
- People learn from their mistakes.
- What may be a heavy investment in training now pays off later.

Complaint management is difficult and takes substantial skill building. As a result, many hospitals with strategies for service excellence use professional trainers to provide training on complaint-resolution skills. However, you can train your own people to develop complaint-management skills and then pass these skills on to the persons who work for them.

If health care organizations want to be the provider of choice when current patients and visitors need future health care, they should also have a squad of people (for example, patient representatives for patients' concerns and a physician liaison for physicians' concerns) who are skilled in complaint resolution and who are able to confront the complaint on a moment's notice. These people should be accessible at all times. Further, they should be invested with the clout needed to elicit cooperation across departmental lines, and they should have time for extensive full-time involvement in handling problems. Even better, the hospital should have a squad of people who interact with the patients, family, and physicians early in their experience and smooth their way through the maze of people, systems, and practices that are typical of most hospitals.

The hospital should also have a group of people whose only job is to handle complaints and who can therefore document and track problems, see patterns, and then facilitate problem solving and actions that prevent these problems from recurring in the future. These staff members may have various titles: *patient representatives, patient advocates,* or *ombudspeople.* The name may be unimportant, but the job they perform is not. No hospital can afford not to have such people. A hospital that has no patient representatives has a painfully acute case of top-management myopia.

☐ Systems Problems

In hospitals especially, systems problems are so critically important in the context of your strategy for service excellence that they deserve special attention. Consider the following example: Rosie started out enthusiastic about our customer relations strategy because she entered health care to help people. She was delighted when the administrators decided to pay attention to the human ingredient in an explicit way. Rosie did all she could to ease long waits in physical therapy: she apologized for delays, kept people posted, offered tea and magazines, and apologized again when the patient was still not seen. Finally, Rosie got fed up: "Why doesn't management fix the scheduling so that people don't have to wait in the first place? Why do I have to spend all my time and energy apologizing to people who are rightfully impatient, bored, and upset because they've been sitting here for hours?" Rosie is right. Rosie has wonderful people skills but is ready to pull the plug on the light she brings to patients because she's so angry about the systems problem that makes her job feel nearly impossible.

An overt attack on systems problems has to be part and parcel of the formula to achieve customer satisfaction and service excellence. Systems problems are not a thing apart. Doing all you can to solve systems problems makes it possible for employees to extend excellent people skills to your customers. In the long run, smooth, user-friendly, and sensible systems are an absolute prerequisite to any sound strategy for service excellence.

Take the test in figure 8-2 while thinking about your organization. "Yes" answers indicate forces already working toward the prevention or solution of debilitating systems problems. "No" answers suggest forces that are interfering with your organization's ability to pave the way for patient satisfaction, physician ease of practice, and employee productivity and satisfaction.

When you have performance problems, your people are doing things wrong. When you have systems problems, your people are doing the wrong things. Your goal is to get people to do the right things right.

George Labovitz, consultant on productivity and quality in health

Figure 8-2. Self-Test: How Effective Are Your Organization's Systems?

Systems Management. Circle the appropriate answer. The more "yes" answers, the better. "No" answers indicate areas that need improvement.

1. Your systems are examined regularly to see if they can be made more user friendly. Yes No

2. Generally, the admissions process runs smoothly without long waits. Yes No

3. Generally, the discharge process runs smoothly without undue confusion or unexpected waits. Yes No

4. Generally, in-house transport services run smoothly, without unexplainable patient waits or equipment shortages that cause undue delays. Yes No

5. Your employees are generally tolerant of systems problems in your facility because they're aware of management's determination to make things run smoothly. Yes No

6. You have effective ways to tackle systems problems that involve many departments simultaneously. Yes No

7. Generally, your systems work smoothly enough that employees don't have to apologize endlessly for systems problems and breakdowns. Yes No

8. Your organization periodically examines those services with the greatest effect on consumer satisfaction to see if it can improve them. Yes No

9. In your organization, service areas are in a logical physical relationship to one another from the customer's standpoint. Yes No

10. Generally, people can get from place to place in your facility without getting too frustrated. Yes No

11. Your billing and collections systems tend to be accurate and problem free. Yes No

12. Forms, items, and other things rarely get lost as they're sent from department to department. Yes No

13. In your organization, decisions get made in a timely fashion. Yes No

(continued)

Figure 8-2. *(continued)*

---

14. In your organization, managers at every level actively accept responsibility for debugging systems problems even when these problems involve other departments.   Yes   No

15. Responsibility for problems is clear in your organization; it is not allowed to ricochet from person to person and from department to department.   Yes   No

Total: __   __

---

care, points out that it costs $1 to fix a problem during the process, $10 to fix it at the end of the process, and $100 to fix it when it reaches the customer. He goes on to claim that the cost of systems problems in service organizations is at least 30 percent of gross sales.

In health care, the cost of systems problems is probably higher. Systems problems cost the organization more than the steps needed to improve them. Reputation problems, denied reimbursement, lawsuits, and staff energy diverted into complaint handling, slow receivables, staff turnover, retraining, access barriers, lost records, and the like are notoriously expensive.

Then, why don't hospitals just fix the systems? They don't because fixing them is tough. George Labovitz tells this instructive joke: A police officer sees a Volkswagen going 50 miles per hour in a 40-mile zone. He also sees a Ferrari going 110. The officer stops the Volkswagen and writes out a ticket. The driver says, "Why me? That Ferrari was going more than 100." The officer replied, "Yeah, but I couldn't catch him."

Blaming customer dissatisfaction on employee behavior is like catching the Volkswagen. You can "catch" employee behavior, but "catching" systems problems is much harder even though systems problems are more likely to play havoc with the long-term satisfaction of every customer. If you ask your employees, your doctors, and your patients what's getting in the way of your hospital being the best it can be, they'll tell you in no uncertain terms: systems problems that go on year after year and oppress everyone.

The Problem: Two Examples

Imagine a hospital in which all staff members excel in people skills. Everyone's gracious, respectful, and sensitive to the needs of patients, visitors, and colleagues. But the hospital is plagued by systems problems. Further imagine that you're a patient at this hospital. When you arrive at the appointed time to be admitted, you're made to wait two hours (because your room isn't ready). You're diabetic, and your doctor made the appropriate diet arrangements, but when your first meal arrives, you can't eat it (because the instructions were fouled up in the kitchen). The next day, both you and your doctor are informed that your test results won't be ready for another 24 hours (because of a miscommunication in the lab). When the results do come back, they are fortunately negative, and you're all set to be discharged. Then you discover a charge on your bill for anesthesia in connection with surgery you didn't have. After an hour's runaround, you finally get the bill straightened out. Despite the fact that everyone at the hospital was genuinely apologetic about these problems and went out of their way to correct them, you vow never to return to this hospital again and make it a point to warn your family and friends.

Now imagine being an employee at the hospital. You work in billing and constantly have to cope with patients whose bills are incorrect. You also have to work with a monstrous computer system and with supervisors who insist that you keep smiling. After months and months of consistent errors that seem inherent in the billing system itself, your patience is gone and so is that of your peers, and you don't care at all about the model people skills that the hospital told you about just a few months ago.

Both these examples show that systems problems are important issues in achieving service excellence.

Obstacles to Improving Systems

Although the causes of systems problems vary from organization to organization, several obstacles to improving them seem universal, particularly among large institutions. Identifying these obstacles is the first step in overcoming them:

- *Acquired myopia.* Recognizing that systems problems even exist is often hard. After people have been with an organization for a few years, they tend to become acclimated to the environment and its ways of doing things. For example, if locating a wheelchair at a given hospital usually takes 20 minutes, a 20-minute wait becomes accepted as normal rather than being attributed to an intolerable scarcity of wheelchairs. A fresh perspective is needed to break myopic reactions and habits.
- *Diffusion of responsibility.* By their nature, most systems problems involve several departments, not to mention many, many people.

Who's responsible? Everyone involved, and that's an obstacle. If everyone has, say, a 5 percent share of responsibility for the system, and therefore the problem, no one person has the authority or control to take the initiative and effect a solution.

- *Territorialism.* Because systems problems transcend departmental boundaries, a lot of finger pointing often results. People tend to see the problem, and the responsibility for solving it, as someone else's; and department heads tend to defend and protect their own people.
- *Complexity.* Once systems problems are acknowledged and a decision is made to address them, their sheer complexity can be overwhelming. Discerning the causes can be difficult and frustrating; implementing a one-shot cure-all can be impossible. Consequently, the commitment to solve the problems often languishes because no solution solves every aspect of the problem.
- *Remote problem solvers.* When responsibility for systems troubleshooting is assumed by top management alone, solutions may be a long time coming because administrators don't have to grapple with the problems on a day-to-day basis. Also, administrators may design elegant solutions that never get refined to levels that are practical and that work. Input is needed from the people who actually implement the systems.
- *Lack of follow-through.* Early success in systems problem solving is often accompanied by a gradual abandonment of the effort. Progress may be followed by progressive complacency so that the problems get only half-solved or the solutions only half-implemented.

Institution of Changes

If any of this sounds familiar, take heart. Isolating the obstacles is half the battle. What follows are methods for overcoming these obstacles:

- *Systems audit.* Before systems problems can be solved, they must be defined clearly. Many consultants specialize in doing exactly that. These consultants conduct systems audits, which are comprehensive examinations of every facet of a troubled system, to ascertain causes and generate options for redressing them. These options in turn suggest who the key players are in creating and executing solutions.
- *Problem-solving facilitators.* Systems problems go beyond the job of one person or one department. By developing a squad of problem-solving facilitators, the organization can delegate the responsibility for mobilizing the right people with a share in the problem and managing the process and group interaction until workable solu-

tions are generated. For such a system to work, the problem-solving facilitators must be empowered with the training and authority to move the group to success.

- *Interdepartmental problem-solving groups.* The easiest way to avert interdepartmental infighting is to set up interdepartmental problem-solving groups. Management insistence on results from these teams forces cooperation. Through such team efforts, divisiveness can transform into synergy.
- *Focused agenda.* Because systems problems are intrinsically complex, no one should expect overnight or perfect solutions. However, incremental improvements can be attained, and they should be the goal. By working through an agenda that focuses on one facet of the problem at a time, the group can achieve ongoing progress and thus feel encouraged, not discouraged.
- *Employee and physician involvement.* Wars are won not only in planning bunkers but also in the trenches. Problem solving depends on the contributions of administrators and managers working with employees and physicians. The participation of employees and physicians through meetings and committees is vital.
- *Feedback mechanisms.* Patient questionnaires, postdischarge telephone surveys, employee and physician surveys, and the watchful eyes of patient representatives and focus groups are all essential in monitoring the progress, or regression, of problem-solving efforts. The feedback thus gleaned can also help detect emerging inadequacies and nip them in the bud, preventing them from being so-called solutions that in reality made matters worse.
- *Appoint a systems problem czar.* A respected manager who is appointed to a two-year term should be given one priority: to solve systems problems with the variety of resources available to the organization. This problem czar makes sure that top management issues a clear, ambitious, and strong problem-attack policy that pushes the czar and everyone who works with him or her to get off the dime and move those mountains. Persistent tough talking is called for. The czar and the employees that he or she works with should have the four T's available: training, tools, time, and a team to help. You have to give the problem czar time because old habits are hard to break.

□ Final Suggestions

Once you gather information about customer satisfaction and complaints, you need to funnel this input into clear mechanisms for figuring out what in the world to do. These mechanisms need to, at various times, involve top management, middle managers, and supervisors, all employees, and a dedicated squad of patient representatives. To the extent that you harness the power of these people to prevent and handle problems and complaints effectively, your organization will cultivate a loyal following that praises you for your responsiveness to their concerns and your concern for their comfort and well-being.

Ask yourself the following questions:

- What are you already doing to solve problems and handle complaints?
- How are your current systems working and not working?
- What alternatives can you consider that would strengthen these systems?
- What priorities have to be identified if needed change is to occur?

In examining your problem-solving, complaint-management, and operational systems, watch for these attitudes, which should be red flags that signal the existence of problems:

- *"Informal problem solving just doesn't seem to work."* Many administrators claim that they listen to complaints, review findings from customer and employee surveys, and keep the findings in mind as they set their priorities. Those methods alone don't solve problems. You must have formal systems for problem solving and complaint resolution so that problems and complaints *systematically* are reviewed and processed. They must not be permitted to fall through cracks.
- *"Complex systems for problem solving are overkill."* The best formal problem-solving systems are simple. For example, once a week, five people sit around a table and read through the complaints of the week and then assign follow-through responsibilities. At their next meeting, they review what happened since. You might try a straightforward quality-circle format. *Simple* systems are more realistic than the fancy, technological systems that require sophisticated project management and tracking techniques.
- *"Results win over processes."* Some people think that a problem has to be processed by committees and more committees, teams and more teams. The result is that the problem is processed to death, and no solutions occur within this lifetime. Many problems can be solved by one person if the culture permits this and trusts its members to make a move without layers of bureaucratic review. In your organization, do people have the authority to solve problems without having to get three layers of approval? If the higher-ups do

not approve of a decision that was made, can the people who made it expect to be forgiven or reprimanded?

- *"Innovation is too risky."* To speed up the problem-solving mentality in your organization, you need to allow more mistakes. Hospital cultures have characteristically discouraged decision making among their managers because it involves taking a risk. Consequently, no decision making or decision by default has become a norm. Are people in your organization afraid that if they try a solution to a problem and it proves unworkable, they will be belittled or punished? If so, why should they bother? If you really want innovation, you have to be willing to accept mistakes from people who are tying to improve the system.

The point to remember about problem solving and complaint management is that if you do not plan to channel the information gathered from your various customer groups about their perceptions of your services into an aggressive, determined problem-solving process, then you shouldn't bother gathering the information in the first place. The hospitals that survive in the challenging years ahead will be those that can unstick themselves from the methods that were used in the past but may not work now and create systems that serve every one of the organization's customers.

Downward Communication

- "They think we're too dumb to understand."
- "Everyone knows but me."
- "Nobody ever tells me anything."
- "What are those guys doing up there anyway?"
- "Who cares. They think we're nobodies."

These laments from employees are frequently the result of inadequate downward communication from administration, from department heads, from supervisors, from the governing board, indeed from every layer perceived as having power and a monopoly on information. A terrific need exists for downward communication. In an information vacuum, employees feel alienated and resentful of administration and rightly so. Why, they wonder, are employees expected to get on the service excellence bandwagon and do all they can for the organization when they are not "let in" on its objectives, challenges, and plights. If administrators claim, "This is your hospital, and you are this hospital," then they should keep employees informed even when there is no big news. Downward communication is essential because it:

- Builds commitment, investment, and ownership.
- Gives people information on which to base their decisions and actions.
- Shows caring and respect for employees. It says, "We know you're there, and we know you care."

Before reading further, take the self-test in figure 9-1. "True" answers show that you're on the right track. "False" answers suggest possible directions for revamping downward communication so that it supports and advances your strategy for service excellence. Then continue reading this chapter to get some helpful suggestions.

□ Communication Fallacies

Just as a person gets arteriosclerosis, organizations get "infosclerosis," hardening of the communication arteries. Organizations become afflicted with infosclerosis because higher-ups in many health care organizations fall victim to six fallacies:

- *Fallacy 1: Thinking no news means no need to communicate.* No news is news. If management fails to communicate about inactions or tabled problems, employees become paranoid, believing either that something has happened and everyone knows but them or that nothing has happened because management has not even *heard* the problem. If people are not told about inactions on a special project, they are convinced that information is being deliberately withheld.
- *Fallacy 2: Thinking that a problem must be 100 percent solved before it becomes news.* What problem in a hospital is ever 100 percent solved? Most solutions are incremental and are only slight improvements in complex systems. However, even slight improvements are news, and administrators should not be ashamed to talk about them. You should inform employees when the process of exploring possible solutions to a problem is begun, even when no one knows if a solution is remotely possible. A process may take years to complete, and yet steps along the way are certainly noteworthy. Employees and physicians can wait a long time for a solution when they know that some action, no matter how slight, is being taken.
- *Fallacy 3: Thinking news has to be big.* Tidbits are big bits to some people. Small bits of news, even such small bits as the repair of the cafeteria's ice machine, deserve air time. If you communicate all the little things, employees are more tolerant of the difficulties involved in solving the big problems. Administrators then feel less desperation and pressure about making the big things happen.
- *Fallacy 4: Thinking employees should hear only good news.* Administrators should not act like overprotective parents. Employees resent this attitude: "Do they think we're too immature or weak to handle bad news and help our organization cope with it?"
- *Fallacy 5: Assuming middle management is an effective funnel.*

Figure 9-1. Self-Test: How Good Is Your Downward Communication?

Downward Communication. Circle the appropriate answer. The more "true" answers, the better. "False" answers indicate areas that need improvement.

1. Your employees at all levels are informed about your organization's financial situation and competitive position.   True   False

2. Your employees at all levels are generally aware of the new challenges that health care organizations face and the strategies under way in your organization to tackle these challenges.   True   False

3. Your employees are generally aware of their importance in attracting patients.   True   False

4. In your organization's "image" materials, for example, annual report and employee and patient handbook, your high priority on customer satisfaction is stated and restated to reinforce its importance in your culture.   True   False

5. Your house publications carry features on customer relations issues, events, and accomplishments.   True   False

6. You have a system for updating your employees on the economic challenges ahead for your organization, so they know how and what you are doing.   True   False

7. When administrators tell middle managers to communicate certain news downward, you can be reasonably certain they will convey it to their subordinates.   True   False

8. Your top management keeps people posted about problems that have been solved.   True   False

9. Your top management admits it when they are not going to devote time and attention to solving a specific problem.   True   False

10. Your top management tells employees when problems and projects are in the midst of being explored even if there's no particular progress being made on them.   True   False

                                         Total: ____ ____

Alas, department heads don't always hear what top management says, absorb it, and convey it downward to subordinates. Recently, a CEO in one hospital invited employees on all three shifts to a series of open forums. She promoted these opportunities by announcing them to department heads and encouraging them to tell their people about them. She also sent a memo to all department heads and requested that it be posted where employees could see it. After the first forum attracted only eight people, a hallway survey was conducted to see if employees knew about the forum and decided against attending or if they simply didn't know about the forum. The surveyor found that only 2 people out of 43 knew about the forum. This situation is an example of a middle-management logjam, a not uncommon situation. Top management needs to admit these situations exist and do something assertive to break through them.

- *Fallacy 6: Thinking you should only communicate news that makes you look good.* You'll look better by being honest, even if the news isn't good, than by being tight-lipped and hoarding information.

Communication needs to be liquid, flowing down the power hierarchy through systematic, recurring, and habitual channels. Managers and supervisors at each level need to stay in touch with the information needs and concerns of their subordinates, to aggressively seek the information that responds to these needs and concerns, and then to provide information to their people. Also, information that people didn't know enough about to request should also be funneled downward on a systematic, recurring, and habitual basis.

☐ What to Communicate and How

The hallway surveyor mentioned earlier asked 43 people what they wanted to know from higher-ups on a regular basis in order to feel informed about, committed to, and confident in their organization. Although this research is admittedly weak, the results smack of simple truths.

Employees want to know:

- Where is the organization going?
- What vision do the leaders have?
- What values are the leaders (and consequently the employees) being driven by?
- How is the organization doing?

—What's good, and what are the consequences?
—What are the problems and their consequences?
—What is the organization doing to make things better?
● What are employees supposed to do? What's their role in all this?

Employees want to feel that:

● This is their organization, and people on the top know it.
● Everyone's in this together. If people don't hang together, they'll all hang separately.
● The higher-ups hear those below them.
● The higher-ups care about the employees.
● The higher-ups respect the employees.
● The higher-ups rely on the employees.
● The higher-ups appreciate the employees.

In the past, employees were rarely informed about their organization's financial health because this health was taken for granted. However, employees need and deserve to understand the competitive environment and its consequences for their organization if they are to extend themselves to help their facility compete successfully. After all, if their organization thrives, their jobs are secure. If their facility's financial health deteriorates, their jobs and futures are threatened. Figure 9-2 shows an example of a reinforcing letter that one administrator sent to all employees in her organization to convey her vision about service excellence and also to put it into a larger economic context.

Many hospitals, especially those with active strategies for service excellence, recognize the need for *employee updates* as well as written communication. Employee updates are *live* presentations, for example, slide shows, speeches, and discussions held ideally by administrators round the clock for all employees, that are designed to update employees on the organization's health and challenges. Updates are a kind of progress report.

At the University of Missouri-Columbia Hospital and Clinics in Columbia, Missouri, the hospital administration conducts updates using a question-answer format at least twice a year. Figure 9-3 shows how they advertise a forthcoming update. Then, realizing that not all staff can attend the updates, the administration circulates to all staff a clear, complete written communication sharing the questions raised and their answers. Figure 9-4 shows an excerpt from such a communication.

Einstein Medical Center conducts at least annual economic briefings that are more structured. These briefings:

- Summarize the factors causing the shift to acute competition among hospitals.
- Describe the competitive situation of its hospitals and how it is doing in the face of competition.
- Describe the nature and rationale for the array of marketing strategies under way in its hospitals.
- Explore with employees what they can do to help its hospitals compete successfully.

Figure 9-2. Sample of Letter to Employees That Puts Service Excellence into Larger Economic Perspective

---

Report from Administration

Dear Fellow Employees:

In an environment of increased competition, our Division is undergoing change. Although these are challenging times, there is a danger. With so much on our minds and with not enough time to do what we need to do yesterday, there is a risk of neglecting the all important human element—personal touch.

I am concerned that we do not forget the real reason for our hospital's existence—providing quality care to our patients. Unlike us, patients are not thinking about prospective payment or preferred provider organizations or hospital marketing. They only know that they are hurting or that they are scared. Although we are familiar with the hospital environment, most patients are not. We must strive to be aware that they may be seized with fright when faced with cold machines and cold voices.

As a hospital, we have much at stake. Hospital care is turning into a "buyer's market." Patients are, and for good reason, choosy about which hospitals they use. The advantage lies with the hospital whose employees are seen as friendly, sensitive, understanding, generous with time, compassionate, and attentive. I want our hospital to pursue that advantage.

In the last two years, we have made terrific gains in the HOSPITALity we extend to our patients and visitors. Although the pressures on us are greater than ever, I know that together we will meet the challenge, become distinguished for our HOSPITALity, and strengthen the quality of care and service we extend to our friends and neighbors. I believe we are special, and I want to get the word out.

During the last few months, you were asked to participate in several programs to reinforce and advance our HOSPITALity effort. I am enthusiastic about these programs and hope you found them stimulating and worthwhile to attend.

Thank you for your active cooperation and for giving our hospital your best.

A. Susan Bernini
Vice-President and General Director
Albert Einstein Medical Center,
Northern Division

Figure 9-3. Announcement of a Forthcoming Information Update

EXTRA
★★★★★

Hospital Headlines

| Vol. 1 No. 2 | UMC Hospital and Clinics | April, 1987 |

STAFF UPDATES!!

UMCHC staff invited to discuss hospital topics in open forums on Thursday, April 30

The Staff for Life urged to bring questions for hospital administration

M105 is Update Site.

Shuttle to be operated from Rock Quarry Center for Staff Updates in M105

Mr. Smith and administrative staff to present program on varied topics. Question-and-answer session follows

Staff Update schedule varied to accommodate staff

(TSFL) Columbia—To ensure staff members working all shifts have an opportunity to attend a Staff Update, a day-long schedule for Updates has been established.

TIME	LOCATION
6:00- 7:15 a.m.	M105
8:30- 9:45 a.m.	M105
10:15-11:30 a.m.	Rock Quarry Center
12:30- 1:45 p.m.	M105
2:00- 3:15 p.m.	M105
4:00- 5:15 p.m.	M105
6:30- 7:45 p.m.	M105

Reprinted with permission of the University of Missouri-Columbia Hospital and Clinics in Columbia, Missouri.

151

Figure 9-4. Excerpt from a Published Communication after an Update Session

---

Staff Benefits

Q Do we have any plans for paying staff members for unused sick days?

A A proposal for this, prepared by the hospital Personnel department, is currently under consideration at the University of Missouri level. The proposal would allow payment to staff members for a portion of the unused sick-leave days. The issue has been made a priority for the hospital this year. Since it would affect all campuses of the University, the proposal must be approved by the University of Missouri.

Q Will there be a change in the rules so staff members can use sick time for sick kids?

A Staff members can now use four days of sick leave to care for ill family members. If more days are needed, supervisors may authorize staff to use personal days or vacation days.

Parking

Q Can staff members park in the garage if they have a meeting at the hospital?

A Not at this time. Patients have the first priority for using the garage. Right now the garage is busy enough that it must be reserved for patients and visitors.

Food Service

Q Why does the cafeteria close at 7 p.m.?

A Business declines dramatically after 7 p.m., and cafeteria administration decided to close it. But after listening to staff input, the administrators decided to reopen the cafeteria from 8 p.m. to 3 a.m.

Professional Services

Q Assuming we are a nonprofit organization, why can't we have a profit-sharing program with staff members?

A By law we can't. Federal tax law prohibits profit sharing in a strict sense for not-for-profit organizations.

Reprinted with permission of the University of Missouri-Columbia Hospital and Clinics in Columbia, Missouri

Following are more vehicles for getting the word out:

- If your organization is going through construction, renovation, or a move, put out a facilities update.
- Put tent cards on cafeteria tables.
- Have your administrator convene an *Opinion Leader Committee* and give the committee regular updates. This action ensures that the word gets spread naturally through your organization's grapevine.
- Set up a *Speakeasy* in which 10 employees have breakfast or lunch with the CEO and discuss what's going on.
- Establish a *direct-line phone information service.*
- Start a *Speaker's Bureau on Hot Projects.* The speakers are members of the administrative team who are willing to speak on individual projects at department meetings.
- Have your customer relations coordinator *interview a service department head* each week and publish the interview in the hospital's newsletter.
- Put a *Daily Slice of Life* (a news brief) on your TV system if you have one.
- Put *graffiti* on toilet walls (no, not lipstick or magic marker, but signboards).
- Post *bulletin boards* along waiting lines in the cafeteria.
- Post *key indicators* (for example, number of admissions and average length of stay) daily for all to see. Examples of places to post the key indicators are in staff bathrooms and lounges.
- Set up quarterly *rap sessions* with the CEO and publish the highlights of these sessions and circulate them to all employees.

☐ Downward Communication of Complaints and Suggestions

Many management teams make a common practice of inviting employee and physician complaints and suggestions. Suggestion boxes, focus groups, employee surveys, and all the other tools described in the discussion in chapter 7 produce reams of complaints and suggestions.

Most employees feel valued and respected when they are invited to participate. They think that "the powers that be care what I think." However, this glow only lasts if management *responds.*

Too often many managers deflect, deny, or ignore the message. Imagine this statement sent to you by an employee: "Many employees are upset about rumors of layoffs." Here are typical management responses that turn off employees:

- *Deflecting:* "Rumors happen everywhere, no matter what's happening. They don't mean much."
- *Denying:* "You really can't let things like this get to you."
- *Ignoring:*No response.

Instead, managers should respond to employee inquiries and comments, either agreeing or rejecting them:

- *Agreeing:* "I realize you're upset. I would be too. We'll look into this and get back to you with the straight scoop."
- *Rejecting:* "I realize you're upset. However, I've been assured that no layoffs are about to happen."

The *worst* response is *no response.* When no one responds to employees, they feel cheated, set up, devalued, ignored, and consequently resentful. To avoid the communication-gap trap that develops when you invite employees to submit ideas and then you communicate nothing further:

- *Respond in writing.* You can't depend on a small group of people (for example, department heads and other managers) to communicate accurately to *all* employees. Messages get lost and mixed up: remember how quickly information got distorted or lost in the old "telephone" or "whispering down the lane" games.
- *Respond in a timely fashion.* Employees need *responses,* not necessarily *solutions,* and they need them quickly so they don't think you've forgotten about them or ignored their ideas.
- *Respond to all suggestions.* Employees need to know that their input is important and that what may be small suggestions to improve daily work life are just as important to the organization as larger ones. Respond, even if you don't adopt the ideas.

Of course, when you ask for employee input, you often get a lot more than you want or need. Here's a method for categorizing an onslaught of ideas and complaints from employees so you can respond in a systematic fashion:

- Step 1: Categorize all of the ideas and complaints. For example, are the ideas or complaints "environmental" or "technical"? Do they relate to problems with "systems," "people skills," "amenities," or "programs or services"?
- Step 2: Pick one category and classify each item in that category using the following scheme:
  —"We've already done something about that." (Perhaps you've

already solved that problem or fixed the broken item but never told anybody that it was taken care of. Communicate that information now.)

— "We know that's a problem, and here's our plan for addressing it."
— "We didn't know that was a concern. Now that we do, here's our plan for looking into it."
— "We know that's a problem, but we can't do anything about it now. Here's why."

- Step 3: Write a memo and distribute it to all staff. Use paycheck stuffers, a column in your in-house newsletter, or any other method to reach *all* employees. Don't rely only on verbal communication to small groups of employees. Your responses won't reach everyone.

Frequent and honest downward communication in response to employee complaints and ideas keeps employees motivated and thinking on your organization's behalf. *Ask, listen, and respond.*

☐ Downward Communication about Service Excellence

As you move forward implementing piece after piece of your strategy for service excellence, communicate with employees about each step of the implementation process, as well as people's reactions to that step, and the plans that emerge from the reactions. This communication helps keep service excellence in the forefront of peoples' consciousness.

If you invite employees to sound off about your organization's service strengths and weaknesses, publish these comments and administration's response to keep communication ongoing. Figure 9-5 shows an example of such a response.

In your employee publication or in a special customer relations publication, include a customer relations feature on such topics as:

- The number of people attending your systemwide workshops so far
- The names of the workshop leaders and their experiences as workshop leaders
- News reports on employee reactions to the workshops
- Evaluation results that include employee, physician, and patient perceptions of employee behavior
- A feature on administrators' reactions to attending numerous sessions and what they learned
- A thank-you from the CEO to everyone for the strains the staff endured and the cooperation they offered one another in order to

Figure 9-5.   Sample of Administration's Response to Suggestions

---

Report from Administration

In response to your steady stream of suggestions, we're continuing to improve our HOSPITALity toward patients. Here's a nutshell summary of recent improvements:

- **Signs** (at last!). The Maintenance Department designed and installed a whole series of directional signs. Hopefully, these make it easier for patients and visitors to find their way and relieve the burden you've carried of answering so many questions and handling so many lost people.
- **Newspapers.** You asked that newspaper boxes be moved inside. We can't because of lobby clutter. But we have arranged for the gift shop and coffee shop to sell newspapers.
- **Free and Available Radio and TV.** In February, we installed two TV channels and two radio stations on every patient TV. One TV channel carries regularly scheduled patient education films. The other will show a clock, advertise hospital services and events, and offer special programs. (Patients still have to pay for access to other TV channels.)
- **Employee Nametags.** Soon, we will be providing you with bold, new nametags that can be read from a distance.
- **Employee Lounges.** You will have lounges. The new buildings and Levy (after renovations) will contain employee lounges on every patient floor and in the OR and lab areas.

If you've submitted a concern or suggestion and haven't heard any response, give me a call at Ext. 6010. We'll do our best to follow up with you if you leave your name and number.

I see steady gains in our HOSPITALity and want to thank you for all you're doing to help.

Sincerely,

Martin Goldsmith

Reprinted from *HOSPITALity News*, Mar 1983, p. 2, Albert Einstein Medical Center, Northern Division, Philadelphia, Pennsylvania

make attendance at the workshops possible
- The major issues raised during the sound-off segments of the workshops
- The status of a few sound-off issues (what's been done, what's being done, what will be done, what can't be done, how interested people can get involved in solutions)

Administrators may also simply report to staff on their perception of the service excellence strategy. This report can be published in the customer relations or employee newsletter or can be sent as an all-staff memo. Figure 9-6 provides an example.

Figures 9-7, 9-8, and 9-9 show examples of other ways to respond to

Figure 9-6. Report on Guest Relations from Administration

Report from Administration

Dear Colleagues,

I am pleased to have this chance to communicate with you about the HOSPITALity program.

Right now we have more than 85% attendance at our HOSPITALity sessions and expect to finish up soon. As you might have noticed, someone from administration sat in on all 55 sessions. It worked out that most of us attended at least six sessions.

As a result, we learned a lot from you ... from your honest, open discussion; from your evaluation forms and from the steady stream of suggestions you've placed in our new suggestion boxes.

Although we'll continue to follow up on your concerns, I want to tell you about a few changes we're making that respond to your concerns:

- In February, we'll have a 24-hour, 7-day-a-week coffee shop, with more seating, new menus, and faster service.
- We're installing "dial discs" on patient phones, so patients can easily call for information, customer relations help, a barber or beautician, a chaplain, etc.
- The main floor public restrooms are on a more frequent cleaning cycle.
- Dietary now sends around a cart that serves early morning coffee.
- We've changed holiday dates in response to the effects our original decision had on your holiday plans.

We're also looking into ways to improve visitor control and security and other big needs you pointed out. We'll keep you posted.

Meanwhile it will take all of our enthusiasm and support to make the HOSPITALity effort a long-lasting success. Together, we can make it happen. I am seeing and hearing many good things. Thank you for all you're doing.

Sincerely,

Martin Goldsmith

Reprinted from *HOSPITALity News*, Jan. 1983, p. 3, Albert Einstein Medical Center, Northern Division, Philadelphia, Pennsylvania

employees. Figure 9-7 shows a form letter to be used when no acceptable solution has yet been found to a problem raised by several employees. Figure 9-8 shows an example of how to report good news to all staff, and figure 9-9 shows an example of how you may pass on to a specific employee a compliment that administration has received from a patient or visitor or physician.

The point is that the printed word, although inadequate by itself, is a must-do vehicle for keeping employees informed. If you circulate substantive information, and not just image-making hype, your readership will steadily increase because people hunger for information that matters.

Figure 9-7. Form Letter for Use in Responding to Unsolvable, but Plaguing, Problems

---

Dear Friends,

I want to get back to you on a problem raised by many employees during our recent workshops on service excellence. People complained about _____, a very complex problem. I agree that this problem has difficult consequences for us, like _____ and _____. With the help of _____ and _____, we've researched possible solutions. Frankly, every possibility that might help the problem seems to lead to several other problems, for instance, _____.

Until we can figure out a way to tackle this problem that doesn't create more problems than it solves, we are not going to take action.

I am asking for your understanding and patience. I am also inviting you to contact _____ to discuss any ideas or approaches you would like us to consider.

Meanwhile, I assure you that we are not forgetting about this problem. It's important, and we know it. I'll keep you informed about any new angles we might decide to pursue.

Sincerely

☐ The "NETMA" Alternative

Want to get even more blatant about your determination to communicate with employees? Consider the powerful *NETMA alternative.* Here's how NETMA works:

- Start by holding a contest in which you ask people to guess what "NETMA" stands for.
- When you have numerous entrants in the contest, write your first *NETMA News* with the opening: "OK, now that we have your attention, we'll tell you what NETMA stands for: "Nobody Ever Tells Me Anything." Then tell your employees and physicians the real scoop about what's going on in your organization at frequent intervals.

Ideally, the *NETMA News* is issued weekly but, if not weekly, then at least at clearly stated, regular intervals. The *NETMA News* is not fancy, but it does the job. It's essentially a typewritten news release with tidbits of news in it.

Why NETMA? Employees have a knee-jerk perception that they are

Figure 9-8. Report Good News to All Staff

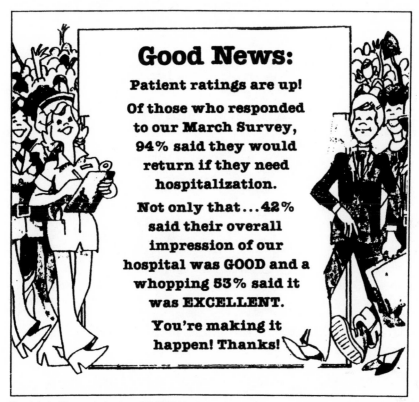

Good News:

Patient ratings are up!

Of those who responded to our March Survey, 94% said they would return if they need hospitalization.

Not only that...42% said their overall impression of our hospital was GOOD and a whopping 53% said it was EXCELLENT.

You're making it happen! Thanks!

Reprinted with permission from *HOSPITALity News*, July 1983, p. 4, Albert Einstein Medical Center, Northern Division, Philadelphia, Pennsylvania.

Figure 9-9. Conveying a Compliment

Look at the great letter from a patient that got directed to me.

(Add complimentary letter or note or memo.)

You did it! <u>You</u> deserve to know about it. I'm so grateful for the honor you're bringing to us through your daily acts of care and compassion.

always uninformed. By calling your news bulletin NETMA and making a "big thing" of it, you confront employees' broken-record gripe that "nobody ever tells me anything." You create dissonance in them and stand the chance of overturning their knee-jerk, and now clearly false, perception. Also, this written piece presses employees to acknowledge that the leadership is taking active steps to keep employees at least partially in the know.

☐ Downward Communication in a Multihospital System

Keeping managers at every level informed about and committed to the multihospital system's mission and priorities is an extraordinary challenge. Barry Brown, chief executive officer of the West Jersey Health System in New Jersey, created the *Corporate Open Forum* to help his people stay in the know. Here's how it works:

- All corporate officers meet as a group with the entire management staff of each of their four hospitals, one hospital at a time.
- The CEO presents a brief update on major initiatives in the system.
- All corporate officers then form a panel and field questions and complaints about anything and everything managers raise.
- Afterward, a social hour encourages further open exchange and team building.

The message conveyed in these corporate open forums is:

- We think of employees in terms of "we" and not "they."
- We're one, a whole, and not fragments.
- You may not see the leadership often, but we're here and we're doing our best.
- We respect your need to know because you are our organization.

The point, in short, is better downward communication by every possible means. The result is improved morale, a better informed work force that has information, not hearsay, guiding their actions and a work force more likely to climb aboard your service excellence bandwagon.

☐ Final Suggestions

Convene a group of influential, informed people to consider together your existing downward-communication practices, their effects, and possibilities for improvement. Then, make decisions and implement them.

The following is a possible process to use with your key people:

- Find out what formal and informal methods you are already using to ensure a downward flow of communication.
- Examine how each existing vehicle is working. Don't guess. Ask employees.
- Identify gaps and needs.
- Generate alternatives. What else might be done?
- Check out the do-able options with your target groups.
- Identify changes you want to make.
- Make the changes. Specify a trial period.
- Evaluate the changes after your trial period.
- Refine the changes based on what you learned during the trial period.

When considering your systems for downward communication, keep the following suggestions in mind:

- *Watch out for one-way communication.* Ensure that communication flows in both directions, from the bottom up and from the top down. Communication is a two-way street.
- *If it's important, then devote time to it.* Delegation of the downward communication job is fine to a point. However, top management needs to personally deliver top-down communication occasionally if they too want to be perceived by workers as credible and concerned.
- *The medium is the message.* Consider carefully the style of both oral and written communications. The style is at least as important as the content. Be frank, empathetic, and human. The following style tips should help:
  —Make communication personal; own what you say. For example, say "I'm concerned about," not "There is concern about."
  —Use feeling words, for example, "I'm worried," or "I'm excited to hear."
  —Be assertive. For example, "I need everyone to do even more" or "We cannot afford to slip now!"
  —Show empathy. "I understand that everyone's feeling the pressure of leaner staffing, and I recognize that people are working very hard, but . . . "
- *Better late than never, but better early than late.* Get information to people quickly. You can be sure employees and physicians will

fume if they read about their organization in the newspaper or hear about it from friends before anyone on the inside spilled the beans.

- *Not just employees, not just the docs.* Some organizations do a great job of communicating to the doctors and insult employees by communicating considerably less to them. The opposite happens in other places. The point is to install timely, regular, forthright communication vehicles that reach both groups.
- *"I said it. Why didn't they hear it?"* Occasionally, check out the absorption rate of what you're communicating. Keep evaluating whether your vehicles for downward communication are *reaching* the right ears.
- *"That's what our public relations department is for."* Your public relations people can help you, but they don't really have their finger on the pulse of employees. The leadership has to take considerable responsibility in identifying news that needs to be communicated and using whatever or whomever to help them communicate it.
- *Be careful of communication overkill.* Whether such a thing as communication overkill actually exists is debatable. However, in case it does, remember to hit the main points in manageable segments. Your communication vehicles have to be carefully honed to help people see the forest through the trees. To check that you've presented the essence, be sure to answer these three questions:
  —What? (the news)
  —So what? (Why am I telling you this?)
  —Now what? (Here's what I'm going to do, and here's what I want you to do.)
- *"What will the neighbors think?"* Adopting the mind set of your target group is vital when you're preparing your communication. How will what you have to say look to the public? Don't get gun-shy and clam up because of possible public perceptions. Just *consciously* fashion the optimal way to get your message across.

Most administrators say that key information eventually filters downward, but according to employees, the filter is often opaque. You need to be more certain that information reaches all employees. You can ensure that communication is indeed reaching people if you have a "healthy" mix of methods for communicating down, up, and across your organization. The result of a good communication system is trust among employees, increased commitment to help the organization succeed, and appropriate, relevant actions enlightened by fact and the respect you've demonstrated toward employees by making sure they have the correct information.

Staff Development and Training

Training is necessary because some people don't know how to act in an *excellent* manner toward guests. Most people do know how to be inoffensive or even good. Excellence, however, requires the seizing of opportunities.

Training helps people recognize opportunities for excellence and develop the skills needed to capitalize on them. It also does more. Training helps people to identify less than wonderful behavior. If you don't train your people in the skills you really value, you'll never know if they wouldn't or couldn't do what you wanted. When you provide training opportunities, you can make this determination. Training is also important because people deserve time to polish their skills and build their sense of professional identity.

Before going on with this chapter, take the self-test in figure 10-1 to evaluate your organization in terms of its employee training systems. Of course, the more "yes" answers, the better. However, "no" answers indicate areas that need follow-up if your strategy for service excellence is going to succeed.

This chapter explores the conditions under which training works to build demonstrable skills in customer serivce. It also identifies a rich array of possible directions for building the skills of your employees.

☐ When and Where

You should not begin training until after you've laid the foundation for the successful application of skills learned to the job. People shouldn't be trained to be great until the systems, management style, and job expectations in your organization support greatness. If you don't wait, you'll see a quick fading of the effects of training and conclude that the training didn't work. The training worked, but the environment didn't support it. This point explains why staff development and training is discussed so late in this book.

Training too soon hurts morale. Your good people want to do well on the job. Training for excellence that then goes unsupported frustrates employees and creates attitude problems that are really justified.

Training too soon also consumes resources. These resources typically include time, use of room, refreshments, costs of instructor, planning time, and participant time. The cost of a typical day's training may be as follows:

- 20 participants x 7 hours x average pay of $11 per hour = $1,140
- Food for 20 at $2 = $40
- Instructor salary or consulting fee = $200 to $3,000
- Space use = $80
- Materials for 20 people at $2.00 per person = $40 plus

In addition, other costs, such as time-consuming scheduling, developing materials, prepublicity, registration, short staffing or replacement hassles in the participants' departments, raised expectations, and much more contribute substantially to the cost. Training is not cheap. Your time and money is only well spent if you create the prior conditions for successful training and for successful transfer of training to the job *before* you rush into training.

Not all training should happen in a classroom situation. Sometimes classroom training can seem ethereal, unreal, too disconnected from the job to take hold. Ideally, the most intense training occurs directly on the person's job, one on one, with the novice shadowing the expert, who coaches, provides feedback, and can engage in instant replays of a situation. Ideally, each department head or supervisor should have a list of standard operating procedures for each job just like the ones hotel people have. Job instruction then focuses on implementing these SOPs skillfully.

The pool manager at the Marriott has a list of 14 steps to take to open the pool every morning. This list was developed after study and discussion with the employees who actually do the job and so could help determine the best way to open the pool. A similar process of SOPs should guide customer relations coaching on how to use a telephone effectively, how to ease long waits, and what to do when a patient complains.

☐ An Orientation Kickoff

If you're just starting a formal strategy for service excellence, consider a systemwide, awareness-raising *kickoff* that orients every person in your organization to your priority on customer relations and your plans to achieve service excellence. Do this before you start skill building. If you've already started skill building, then use this kickoff as a refresher, as a way to reinforce your commitment to service excellence.

All employees need to be oriented to your strategy for service excellence through a widely publicized, mandatory session that is repeated during all shifts. Consider having at least one top administrator present at every session to show the importance of this effort and to demonstrate a commitment and presence that encourages employees to take service excellence in general and the session itself seriously. The session should launch or relaunch the priority on service excellence in your organization, introduce or review relevant policies, and through careful program design, enlist employees' energy and cooperation.

To be effective, the session needs to use state-of-the-art adult education and motivation principles. If you have in-house people who can design it, you have an advantage. If not, numerous outside consultants can help. If you do use an outside consultant or program, make sure the program is customized to your specific setting, culture, and issues.

Here are the basics of a successful kickoff:

- Tell employees the truth about why your organization is launching a full-scale strategy for service excellence. Are you motivated by image problems, an economic downturn, fierce competition, internal conflict resulting from staff insecurity and change, or what? Only the whole truth is believable to employees who were not born yesterday. Tell it like it is. If survival is an issue, then explain that if the organization does not survive financially, employees will lose their jobs.
- Describe what your organization is doing to compete successfully in an increasingly competitive environment and indicate that through your strategy for service excellence, you're asking that every employee play a role in helping your organization to not only survive but also thrive.
- Acknowledge employees for the positive role they have always played in providing high-quality care, but emphasize that in these competitive times, everyone can do even more. All employees must do what they can to make your organization distinctive in the

quality of service extended to customers so that the organization can improve its competitive position, image, and pride.

- Emphasize that although employees certainly did not cause any economic problems, they can help solve or prevent them.
- Have employees evaluate your organization's service from their own viewpoints. Use the self-test in figure 10-1. Give people a chance to vent their frustrations about the obstacles to service excellence in their particular workplace. Allow problems to be confronted openly. Acknowledge problems and reassure employees that their views will be channeled to people with the power to act.
- Present concrete behavioral expectations, such as "House Rules," that define what you mean by excellent customer relations. Make these rules clear, unequivocal, required, and applicable to all.
- Present relevant policies and personnel practices that put teeth in your new standards, for example, through job descriptions, supervisory practices, performance appraisal, and commendation systems.
- Tell people your plan for service excellence.
- Ask them to join you by participating fully.

How long does such a kickoff take? The session for *all employees* usually runs 2½ to 3 hours. From then on, training should be targeted to job-specific groups so that you use their time optimally by focusing, not on generic skills, but on the skills that are key to specific positions.

☐ Targeted Training

Generic programs, such as a kickoff, can certainly build a customer-oriented mind set and raise awareness of the behaviors that reflect it. They can also engage employees in activities that sharpen widely needed skills. However, to move people to *excellence* in customer relations and not just to eliminate blatant rudeness or other offensive behavior, staff need help in *identifying and capitalizing on previously missed opportunities in their specific jobs.* An admissions clerk greeting an incoming patient with "Good morning. May I help you?" is acceptable, but it's not excellent. More impressive is the following from the admissions clerk: "Good morning. My name is Sue Martin. Welcome to Community Hospital! May I help you?" People in specific jobs can be doing more to not only meet customer expectations but also to exceed them and thereby truly impress customers with their courtesy, caring, and compassion.

The distance between being good and great in customer relations lies in missed opportunities, and these missed opportunities are the

Figure 10-1. Self-Test: How Effective Are Your Employee Training Systems?

> **Staff Development and Training.** Circle the appropriate answer. The more "yes" answers, the better. "No" answers indicate areas that need improvement.
>
> 1. Your organization offers training programs periodically to upgrade the customer relations skills of all employees.   Yes   No
>
> 2. Your organization offers training programs to upgrade the customer relations skills of job-specific groups (for example, security guards, information desk staff, admissions staff, nurses, transporters, tray delivery people, and billing personnel).   Yes   No
>
> 3. Your organization trains employees who have the most telephone contact to excel in telephone skills.   Yes   No
>
> 4. Your organization trains employees to view complaints as giving them another chance to satisfy customers.   Yes   No
>
> 5. You offer professional renewal programs to help nurses and other employees handle the stress, pressure, and burnout felt by many these days.   Yes   No
>
> 6. Your organization teaches your employees strategies for team building so that problems within groups and between groups are acknowledged and tackled.   Yes   No
>
> 7. Your organization offers required training for middle managers and supervisors so that they know how to hold employees accountable to high customer relations standards, serve as role models, and recognize and reward excellence when they see it.   Yes   No
>
>   Total: __ __

focus of effective targeted training. Targeted training involves job-specific skill building with selected groups whose performance suggests a need for further development. These groups may warrant additional training because they seem to have problems, or perhaps they merit special attention because of their disproportionately great influence on the first and last impression customers form at your doorstep.

For example, the quality of nursing care has an obvious impact on patient evaluations of a facility. Obviously, nurses stand to gain from the emphasis on caring, courtesy, and cooperation that is stressed in any introductory campaign for service excellence. However, nurses face challenges that few other hospital employees face. How can they meet and even surpass the demands for empathy required by their intimate contact with patients shift after shift, hour after hour, patient after patient? How can they best cope with the difficult patient and the difficult doctor?

Nurses are just one example. Every other specialized role, particularly those involving patient contact, has its own set of special problems and opportunities, and each respective role needs to be examined individually.

Of course, you can't tackle the specifics of every special group simultaneously. The number of relevant groups and the need to go beyond the superficial preclude treating them all at one time. The question then becomes, which groups require specific action first? And the answer is: that depends. Each organization has different needs. Perhaps the best way to establish priorities is to let patient survey data guide you. Maybe the data at one facility are positive toward the nursing staff but indicate dissatisfaction with the transport and tray delivery personnel. If so, you start there.

What are the kinds of skills needed to improve the job-specific performance of special groups? Again, the answer depends on the groups in question. To use the example of transporters, ask them to give one another fast stretcher rides so that they can experience for themselves the difference between their job done poorly and done well. For tray delivery staff, create dexterity impairment exercises, for instance, eating with splints on their fingers or with gloves on, so that they become aware of how an arthritic patient eats a meal. The point is that you must examine the nitty-gritty aspects of specific roles. Identify the problems in each job and treat them as opportunities to exceed patient expectations with spectacular behavior.

You can assess needs by using focus groups, think tanks, interviews, observations, analyses of complaints, patient survey results, and the like. You should have an adequate patient feedback system that points you toward the groups that need the most help. If you don't have such a system, focus on the areas with the most public contact and start there: admissions, billing, outpatient services, emergency department, and housekeeping.

The following sections provide ideas on training for specific groups and in specific subject areas. These suggestions are just a smattering of staff development and training needs and possibilities. You must first find out who needs skills, morale boosts, and attention and then develop, or find, appropriate programs that translate your stated priority on customer relations into an actual investment for your staff. These descriptions may expand your own image of the possibilities and in some cases even strike a chord of "Oh yes, we need that." If you have in-house training resources, you can perhaps develop your own training agenda; if not, seek out knowledgeable consultants. However you do it, the key is to match the program to your organization's needs.

Workshop for Administrators

Your top management or administrative team is one key to the success of your strategy for service excellence. They convey values and priorities to the work force, allocate resources, set policy, and establish expectations for the behavior of all employees. A workshop for administrators helps them examine the special roles they need to play to assert their leadership, to inspire cooperation throughout the organization, and to prevent problems that may impede progress. This program helps administrators refine their role in supporting and strengthening high standards and employee energy and involvement.

The workshop should include the following:

- How administrators function as a role model and how they can develop behaviors that employees can look up to
- How to clarify administration's expectations of department heads in terms of service excellence and how to hold department heads accountable for their own and their employees' behavior toward customers
- How to strengthen the organization's problem-solving and communication systems to build morale, identify and solve sticky problems, ease strains on staff, and trigger energetic cooperation with high customer relations standards
- How to increase the recognition and appreciation that flow through the organization
- How to confront and hold accountable the problem department heads whose own behavior and department drag down the organization's image and reputation with customers

Workshops for Middle Managers and Supervisors

The middle-management layer is your organization's internal accountability mechanism for ensuring that employees meet the standards for service excellence. Special attention to the role of middle management and supervisors is a necessity because middle management is often the weakest link in your strategy.

169

Workshop for Middle Managers

To maximize the strength and results of your strategy, your middle management needs to be committed to service excellence and to be effective in their leadership roles. To reinforce high standards of customer relations behavior and hold employees accountable, supervisors and managers need to, first, be role models of excellent customer relations and, second, manage the positive and negative consequences of their employees' behavior.

The workshop should include:

- Defining the middle manager's and supervisor's understanding of their role in making your strategy for service excellence a success
- Articulating their own personal vision of service excellence for their work group
- Building their commitment and accountability
- Strengthening their behavior as role models of service excellence
- Developing skills for clarifying and communicating explicit, behavioral, and job-specific expectations to their subordinates
- Developing practical techniques for giving positive and negative feedback and for coaching employees in necessary skills
- Managing the problem employee and terminating if necessary those who persistently fail to meet the standards for service excellence

Workshop on Effective Downward Communication

The perception "nobody ever tells me anything" demoralizes employees and dampens their dedication and commitment to your strategy for service excellence. Managers, too, get tired of hearing this gripe. This workshop focuses on hands-on techniques for communicating successfully with employees, countering a "nobody ever tells me anything" attitude, and building morale.

The workshop should highlight the following points:

- Determining what employees need to know
- Dispelling the myth of the all-knowing manager
- Maximizing perception, reception, and understanding of information
- Developing creative techniques to keep employees knowledgeable
- Developing simple techniques for written communication
- Using people-to-people or peer-group communication chains
- Establishing an all-out campaign that confronts that "nobody-ever-tells-me-anything" feeling

- Providing specific help on how to communicate bad news while keeping the faith

Workshop on Morale Building

Employees are hard pressed to always keep their chins up and to unfailingly extend patience, courtesy, and compassion to customers, especially with the pressures and insecurities generated by the rapid changes in health care. This workshop examines employee morale because morale can make or break the ability of an organization's work force to exhibit genuine and excellent service for the sake of the customer and the organization.

The workshop should highlight the following:

- Causes of sinking morale
- Telltale signs of poor morale
- Typical managerial responses to low morale and the ripple effects of these responses
- Repertoire of strategies on how to cope with the overall institutional morale and with the morale of administrators, managers and supervisors, and employees

Workshop on Development of Productive, Energetic Teams

"I came to my job with energy and a real feeling that I could make a difference. Now, all I hear is complaining. Everyone seems out for themselves." Skilled managers and supervisors can overcome this all-too-familiar sentiment through a systematic team-building strategy that infuses their people with team spirit and mutual support, the fuel for ongoing service excellence.

This workshop builds practical skills that help work groups increase both their job satisfaction and their productivity. It should highlight the following:

- Identifying team strengths and weaknesses
- Getting team members to give service excellence a chance and try one more time
- Promoting group cohesiveness while bringing out the best in individuals
- Improving group functioning and spirit by using tried-and-true techniques, such as brainstorming, trust building, constructive feedback, and peer recognition
- Developing a team-building action plan

Workshop on Service Management

In today's competitive environment, health care managers are under increasing pressure to manage their departments as service businesses. Successful performance depends on a strong service-oriented mind set and practices to match. This program examines the key elements of service management. It highlights the following:

- Setting standards that push for excellence, not mediocrity
- Achieving user-friendly service systems and practices for patients, visitors, physicians, and coworkers
- Staying close to the customer and effectively managing customer complaints
- Strengthening leadership in today's service age

Workshop on Discipline and Documentation

Problem employees can drag down the most inspiring customer relations standards if they are allowed to continue their less-than-admirable behavior. Good employees giving their all to service excellence wonder, "Why should I sweat for this place, when Hal is allowed to be rude to people day after day, year after year?"

Managers and supervisors need to sharpen their skills for confronting, coaching, and counseling employees on any customer relations behavior that is less than excellent. This program develops the practical skills for challenging problem behavior, achieving conformity to standards, or terminating the employee.

The workshop should highlight the following:

- Resolving mixed feelings about disappointing behavior, as in "After all, doesn't everyone have a bad day?"
- Moving from "attitude" to "behavior"; describing lapses in excellent customer relations in descriptive, behavioral, and performance terms
- Writing sound disciplinary documents so that disciplinary actions stick
- Enacting every stage in a progressive discipline process applied to customer relations behavior
- Using the "broken record" and "fogging" techniques from assertiveness training for handling discussions with resistant employees

Workshops for Nurses

Many nursing staffs have come under the budgetary scalpel. The implications are many. Nurses who have survived layoffs are expected to do more with less: work more shifts, attend more patients, perform a broader range of duties. With the heightened emphasis on service excellence, they're also expected to do their job with greater sensitivity, patience, and empathy. The result is widespread resistance to customer relations strategies among nurses.

Some organizations have money for nurses but can't find nurses to fill jobs. This situation leads to short staffing, burnout, resentment, and frustration. Expected to serve the sicker quicker, the nurse is weighed down by increasing demands, including the responsibility for winning the patient's and the physician's favor.

In this environment, many nurses and their nurse managers vigorously resist their hospital's strategies for service excellence because they view pressure to pamper the customer as cosmetic, superficial, and commercial. Special programs are needed to build nurse manager support for service excellence and to approach the special needs of the staff nurse in special, appropriate ways.

Workshop for the Nurse Manager

Nurse resistance to customer relations strategies may stem in large part from the fact that many nurse managers have not been sufficiently involved in the design or scope of their hospital's approach to service excellence and customer relations. Tailored training is needed to prevent or overcome the resistance of nurse managers and replace it with active, enlightened support.

This workshop shows the big picture of service excellence to give the concept depth and meaning. It then examines the nurse managers' vision of service excellence in tough, everyday situations and provides suggestions for educating their nursing staffs to fulfill this vision. Highlights of the workshop may include:

- Defining service excellence in nursing
- Discussing the conflicts in nursing that lead to a breakdown in service (for example, the multiple demands on nurses and the emotional drain of working primarily with sick people)
- Managing for service excellence, including suggestions for increasing empathy and handling difficult patients and demanding family members

Workshop on Professional Renewal for Nurses

Nurses need substantive help in coping with the emotional challenges and frustrations of their new environment and the new demands being placed on them. Therefore, consider targeting a special component of your strategy for service excellence to help nurses feel more positive about themselves, more in control, and more equipped to avoid negativity and disabling stress. In short, to strengthen your customer relations effort, nurses need a philosophy and tool kit for working happy.

Using her experience with HARMONY, a renewal program for the nursing professional that she codeveloped for the Einstein Consulting Group with Diana Walker, director of nurse development services, Katie Buckley, director of human resources development services, recommends this content for training nurses to cope with their hyperstressful environment:

- Identify patterns of thinking and action that drain energy and undermine a nurse's ability to sustain a positive outlook
- Redirect the interactions between nurses and patients and other staff so that they enhance pride, emotional availability, and sense of accomplishment
- Build skills for gaining a greater sense of control while handling multiple demands
- Examine strategies for working smarter, not harder
- Rekindle the satisfaction inherent in working with and for patients
- Explore healthy ways to handle stress

Assertiveness training for nurses, including how to handle the difficult doctor, and an advanced program stressing more sophisticated customer relations skills are also time well spent to engage nurses in building a repertoire of interpersonal skills that make a difference to customers. Possible items to include in such programs include:

- How to give intense personal attention so that patients and visitors feel special
- How to respond empathically
- How to turn complaints into opportunities to heighten customer satisfaction
- How to deal with the difficult patient and the difficult doctor

The options are many. The important thing is *to do something special for nurses.* Whether you agree or not, you need to be aware that nurses perceive their situation as unique, and consequently, they require special understanding and an especially sensitive approach to help them handle problems with customer relations.

Workshops for Front-Line Employees

All nonsupervisory employees need skill-development opportunities that heighten their motivation with regard to customer relations and their development of sophisticated customer relations skills. Following are descriptions of a smorgasbord of programs that can help accomplish these objectives.

Workshop on Skill Building for Front-Line Employees

A few employee groups repeatedly generate first and lasting impressions of your organization, for example, personnel at the information desk, transporters, tray deliverers, security guards, and housekeepers. These public contact personnel are your front-line people. Inherent in these positions are special problems and special opportunities. The continued effectiveness of your strategy for service excellence depends on reinforcing employees' views of themselves as public contact professionals and strengthening the attitude and skills that optimize your organization's image.

The highlights of this workshop may include:

- Understanding the vital role of front-line people in customer relations
- Identifying key moments of truth in their contacts with your organization's customers
- Creating powerfully positive first impressions
- Developing the verbal and nonverbal behaviors essential to customer satisfaction
- Using initiatives to ease long waits
- Practicing techniques for handling irate customers and other difficult situations
- Understanding the basics of customer-conscious and salesminded telephone communication

You can use a program similar to the one for front-line employees to cultivate positive relationships between your facility and the staff in physicians' offices. This program can also strengthen the customer relations skills and awareness among the physician's own staff.

Workshop on Handling Difficult People

Even those individuals with the best skills and attitudes encounter patients, doctors, and other customers who test their coping abilities to the limit. This workshop builds the skills necessary for handling a wide range of difficult people and situations while maintaining personal emotional health and a professional demeanor. It highlights the following:

- Personal prejudices and preconceptions that make some encounters so difficult
- Control through action, not reaction
- Active listening to uncover hidden meanings
- Step-by-step process for handling the irate person
- Assertive communication of your message
- Nondefensive complaint management
- Strategies to use when you're at your wit's end
- Dissatisfied customers as opportunities to win loyal customers

Workshop on Caring for the Older Adult

Most patient populations include a substantial portion of older adults. Although working with older people raises important clinical questions, it also requires highly developed customer relations sensitivity and skills that reflect the courtesy, dignity, and respect that elderly people, and all people for that matter, deserve and expect from health care providers.

This workshop examines stereotypes of the sick elderly person and builds the special skills and sensitivity required to promote a sense of dignity and independence. The following should be highlighted in this workshop:

- Myths and realities regarding older people
- "Physical-limitation experiments," for example, seeing the world through foggy glasses, eating with gloves on, and walking with stones in shoes, that enable you to identify your own patterns and responses to uncomfortable or disabling situations
- Offensive behaviors as reported by elderly patients, for example being talked to in a condescending manner ("Are *we* ready for our bath?" "Hi, sweetheart, have you been a good boy since I saw you last?")
- Specific interpersonal skills that foster mutual respect, confidence, independence, and an atmosphere of caring

Workshop on Conflict Management

Managers and supervisors spend an inordinate amount of their time resolving conflicts. This time needs to be well spent because time is too valuable to be spent on unproductive problem solving.

This workshop develops skills for productive conflict management so that relationships especially among coworkers are positive and cooperative. It should highlight the following:

- Personal style of handling conflicts and what works for and against you
- Methods of increasing your power to influence others
- Conversion of conflict into positive and constructive resolution
- Communication skills that encourage openness and cooperation in coping with conflicts

Workshop on *Effective Coworker Relationships*

Most health care jobs are stressful enough without having additional stress created by problematic relationships with coworkers. Turning a problem relationship into a relationship that works for both people leads to both successful and satisfying work.

This workshop builds skills and problem-solving techniques that improve those all-powerful day-to-day relationships with coworkers. The workshop should highlight the following:

- Getting what you need from your coworkers
- Communicating to get results
- Resolving conflicts productively
- Negotiating terms in the worst of situations
- Expanding your skill repertoire to enhance your own on-the-job comfort

Workshop on *Practical Assertiveness on the Job*

Many employees are appropriately assertive in the workplace, but some can become overly aggressive or too passive at crucial moments. In this workshop, participants examine the importance of assertiveness in today's workplace and learn to communicate honestly and directly with customers and coworkers. This course is on workplace survival. The highlights of the workshop can include:

- How to handle delicate situations and resolve delicate conflicts
- How to say what you want and think with appropriate tact
- How to develop confidence and take appropriate risks
- How to get cooperation when you need it
- How to say "no" without feeling guilty
- How to handle adverse reactions to your assertiveness without selling out

177

Workshop on Telephone Tact and Tactics

Employees typically reduce their expectations of themselves on the telephone because they feel anonymous. The result is a tarnished organizational image. If a health care organization wants to project a professional image and build goodwill, employees who work with the public need to handle the telephone with skill and sensitivity. Public contact professionals, such as receptionists, secretaries, medical clerks, and telephone operators, need to understand and be understood while at the same time making callers feel cared for and respected by the organization.

This workshop is concerned with the way people handle the telephone: how they answer, how they put people on hold, how they handle the angry or impatient caller. The workshop should highlight the following:

- Making the connection between telephone communication, customer satisfaction, and the organization's image
- Responding with care and tact to the obvious and hidden aspects of a conversation
- Presenting yourself, your boss, and your organization in the most favorable light possible
- Building people's confidence in the organization through impeccable competence and courtesy
- Practicing specific telephone protocols for handling typical daily challenges

Workshop on Making the Most of a Minute

Some employees resist customer relations standards because they don't have time. This workshop is for staff who actually have, or think they have, only fleeting contact with patients, such as tray delivery workers, housekeepers, and maintenance workers. The workshop highlights:

- The impact "moments of truth" have on patients
- Verbal and nonverbal skills that help staff make the most of even small amounts of contact with patients, for example, how to greet patients warmly and how to make the most positive impression in two or three sentences
- A repertoire of impressive customer relations behavior that enables the employee to establish contact with patients without interfering with the work they came to do, for example, having a pleasant facial expression when entering the room and having a few standard

sentences that can be used to acknowledge the presence and importance of the patient

Workshop on Viewing Complaints as a Second Chance

This workshop on viewing complaints as a second chance makes every employee see the importance of empathy as a technique for understanding patients' frustrations. It also covers how to make quick, resourceful responses to patient, visitor, and physician complaints. It emphasizes what employees can do to minimize the number of patients and physicians who "go away mad or just go away." The following can be highlighted in this workshop:

* Complaints as opportunities to develop loyalty to your organization and to get repeat business
* Practice of a step-by-step complaint-handling process that makes escalating conflict nearly impossible:
  —Hearing the person out; encouraging venting in full
  —Showing you understand without having to agree or disagree
  —Apologizing for any distress caused
  —Offering alternatives
  —Following through
  —Thanking the person for speaking up

Workshop on Professional Renewal

Are some people's energy and motivation fading and their enthusiasm for work slipping? This workshop on professional renewal helps people explore their personal gifts, talents, and strengths and gives them practical ways to transform self-imposed limits into new confidence, satisfaction, and energy for work. The workshop can highlight the following:

* Methods for building self-affirmation into your life at work, for example, establishing buddy system reminders or keeping key one-liners on the inside of your locker ("You *are* making a contribution to your patients!")
* Structured experiences that support self-discovery and self-enhancement
* Practical ways to enrich your personal life on and off the job
* A repertoire of stress management tools and practical, easy mind-centering methods, such as visualization, physical movements, and breathing techniques, that you can draw on in the face of job stress and strain

Workshop on Stress and Distress on the Job

Given the multiple demands, heavy workloads, and sensitive inter-personal situations, health care personnel need to devote conscious attention to maintaining their balance in the face of stress, pressure, and competing demands. Otherwise, frustration, burnout, and illness strike.

This workshop goes beyond awareness raising to building a reper-toire of tools and skills that give people some control over their physical, mental, and emotional well-being in the face of a job that is so stressful that distress results. The following can be highlighted in this workshop:

- Stress patterns and where they lead
- Difference between appropriate, productive stress and distress
- Identification of key sources of stress in your life
- The skills grab-bag, including techniques for relaxing, thinking straight, setting priorities, and being assertive when others are the stress source
- Personal action plan for keeping your balance and your health

☐ Customer Relations as a Professional Asset

Consider providing employees with a set of customer relations courses that enable them to earn certification in customer relations. You can, for instance, offer a basic program of required modules, electives, and a supervised "internship." When employees have successfully completed the required combination of program compo-nents, they become certified in customer relations. You can hold certification ceremonies so that other employees, family members, and friends can witness the granting of these customer relations certificates.

This kind of program can be a powerful motivator, especially for the nonprofessional people who have fewer chances to become "creden-tialed" than do nurses and managers. A certification program enhances the message that excellence in customer relations is substantive and takes work. Also, it leads to recognition; to increased self-esteem; to enhancement of the employee's marketability; and better yet to salary increases, promotions, higher grade jobs, or other perks. A certification program is one way to inspire perseverance in developing customer relations skills in the kind of depth that pushes people beyond inoffensiveness to achieve service excellence.

☐ Final Suggestions

The opportunities for training and staff development programs abound. Because training can be expensive in terms of time and energy, consider these tips so that you can see definite results from your training activities:

- *Don't train before you install service excellence as an organizationwide priority.* Whomever you choose to train first is bound to ask, "Why us? Are we so bad?" They think you're singling them out or pointing a finger and in a way, you are. That's why a systemwide orientation is important before you home in on a specific group for skill enhancement.
- *Beware of Band-Aid® skill training.* For example, you determine that your admitting officers are not customer-oriented. They're rude, treat patients as interruptions, move too slowly, and speak in curt tones. The department head calls in your training department or an outside consultant to provide an urgently needed, one-day skill-building program for your admitting officers. The trainer arranges a well-structured, educationally sound workshop that includes such topics as developing the basic skills of meeting and greeting, easing the patient's long wait, making small talk to ease anxiety, and handling complaints. The group loves it because it's a day away from the job, a break in the routine, food for thought. Then they go back.

  All kinds of things may happen that pose barriers to their continued use of the learned skills on the job:
  —They weren't convinced of the value of the skills learned, and the boss doesn't reinforce the importance or the necessity.
  —They try the new skills and fail, and the boss doesn't bother coaching toward success.
  —They don't have a chance to try the new skills, and so they forget them.
  —They try the new skills but get no feedback, and consequently, they lose their confidence and motivation to stretch.
  —They apply the skills well and get punished for it.

  In such cases, you may conclude that the training failed. The training did not fail. The training built the necessary motivation and skill, but it was undermined by actions or sins of omission by their boss and the department's systems when the trainee applied the new skills on the job. Training just cannot work in a vacuum. To reap results, a foundation should be in place that enforces and reinforces the skills learned. That's why upfront work with administrators and the training of middle managers and supervisors is so

181

important as a prior condition of training.

Customer relations coordinators who promise behavioral improvements as a result of short-term training without adequate systems supports are an endangered species. Such Band-Aid™ training at best only treats the symptom and offers no more than short-term relief.

- *Don't be punitive; empower people.* People need to build and apply new skills in an atmosphere of acceptance and motivation.
- *Don't put off training needs until a more convenient time.* What with the multiple demands on people's time and the complexity of scheduling, no time is ever convenient for training. One hospital wanted their ambulatory care staff to do a better job of meeting, greeting, and putting people at ease. Building excellence in the requisite skills takes supervised practice and feedback. The responsible trainer could provide the structure for this training in an intense seven-hour program. However, the hospital people would neither give up their desire to get these people trained nor provide the seven hours. The compromise was a series of three-hour sessions held a week apart. The results were three scheduling hassles instead of one, a skill-building series too diffused to build the professional identity that truly motivates, a program so truncated that little skill practice fit in, and consequently no transfer of skills to the job situation. The cost of the programs was $2,000 in staff time and dashed hopes. If you're going to do training and want results, do an adequate job of it or revise your expectations downward.
- *Don't set your standards too low.* Train for excellence, for impressiveness. Simply eliminating offensive behavior is not enough.
- *Don't leave desirable behavior to people's imagination.* In a recent program, 30 supervisors were divided into groups of 3. Each trio was asked to spend 20 minutes preparing a demonstration of making the most of a small amount of time with a patient, such as delivering a patient tray, changing a light bulb, giving directions in the hallway, or checking the TV. Two of the 10 demonstrations were excellent. Most were mediocre, although inoffensive, but two had offensive elements in them. The trainer had to devote substantial time to helping the groups polish their scenarios to eliminate offensive aspects and tap missed opportunities. A short exercise turned into an all-day activity for good reason. If your managers don't know what excellence looks like in everyday situations, how can they move their people toward it? Excellence is not always obvious, and training programs need to direct the group's attention to defining it in concrete terms for each person's job.
- *Don't overuse scripting.* Some businesses teach a standard script

and require every employee to use it with every customer, the so-called programmed robot approach. In a health care setting, this approach can be fraught with problems:

—Employees don't have to think or feel, and so phoniness is the likely result.

—Customers lose confidence in the organization because it's obvious that employees are not treating or responding to them as individuals. They may not mind such standardization at McDonalds, but in hospitals where they expect and deserve *personal* attention, they mind.

—Employees suffer from terminal tedium. The room for spontaneity and invention in their jobs is limited. The redundancy of the work, a by-product of scripting, shows itself in boredom and listlessness.

That's the downside of scripts, but they also have an up side. Consider scripts as *fallback positions* when employees are in the doldrums. If you have a canned way to act and talk when you're feeling low or upset, that canned approach is probably better than the way you would act if you let your mood dictate your behavior. Also, by seeing that every employee learns at least one "excellence script" for use in the typical situations they handle, you're ensuring that employees understand at least one definition of excellent behavior. You can stretch employees' vision of excellence by working out really great scripts.

To protect yourself against the potential tedium and impersonality of one script that employees use repeatedly, consider developing with your employees a small repertoire of scripts. This action allows for much more choice, employee judgment, and spontaneity and provides a break from perfunctory behavior.

The Japanese recognize that well-trained employees can make or break a company. As a result, Japanese workers typically spend 25 percent of their first six years with a company in various kinds of training programs. Hitachi, an electronics giant, spends more than $80 million a year on employee training. This amount is equal to about two-thirds of the company's advertising budget.

Robert Hayes, a business professor at Harvard University and co-author of *Restoring Our Competitive Edge: Competing through Manufacturing* (New York City: John Wiley & Sons, 1984), says that over the long haul, American managers would be wise to rethink their training strategies if they want to stay competitive. Hayes emphasizes the importance of upfront investments in training to instill the discipline, skills, and pride essential to providing the high-quality services that win consumer favor.

Training must be an inherent, extensive, and ongoing component of your strategy for service excellence if you want to ingrain into your culture the powerful value of customer relations and infuse your people with the requisite skills.

Physician Involvement

One of the most complex challenges in achieving service excellence is how to mobilize the medical staff. The question "what to do about the doctors?" is usually agonizing. Before continuing with this chapter, take the self-test in figure 11-1 to see how involved your physicians are in your strategies for service excellence. The more "yes" answers, the greater their involvement. The real clues to further possibilities are in the "no" answers.

Excellent customer relations on the part of physicians is obviously desirable from your organization's point of view because doctors interact with hospital patients and because nonmedical staff become disgruntled with a double standard. Achieving excellent customer relations is easier when doctors are paid employees, which is a rapidly increasing trend. Paid physicians, like other employees, can more easily be held accountable to internal customer relations expectations. However, most doctors have admitting privileges at several institutions and are themselves customers of the hospital, and so imposing customer relations standards on them is a lot trickier.

Before approaching the doctors, the administration must decide on the level of risk it is willing to assume. Administration must consider whether its doctors are voluntary attending physicians or salaried employees and what degree of customer relations pressure its competitors apply to physicians. The question is whether to treat your doctors as customers, as accountable partners in care giving, or as both. What degree of tact is important to your organization?

Before exploring alternative approaches, let's look at what doctors

Figure 11-1. Self-Test: How Involved Are Your Physicians?

Physician Involvement. Circle the appropriate answer. The more "yes" answers, the better. "No" answers indicate areas that need improvement.

1. Physicians are aware that service excellence is an organizational priority. Yes No

2. Your physicians see themselves as part of your strategy for service excellence. Yes No

3. You've made your physicians aware of the specific behavioral expectations that constitute service excellence. Yes No

4. When a physician violates your standards for service excellence, that physician is confronted in a constructive way. Yes No

5. When your physicians have a complaint, they know whom to call. Yes No

6. You have a clear system for responding to physician complaints and needs. Yes No

7. Influential physicians are involved in strategic planning for service excellence in your organization. Yes No

8. Physicians are not exempt from pressure toward service excellence in your organization. Yes No

Total: ___ ___

---

have to gain from customer relations. After all, if you want your approach to work, it has to appeal to doctors' own needs.

☐ Benefits for Doctors

In your hesitation to impose any demands on physicians for fear of turning them away from your organization, you may not pay adequate attention to the benefits that doctors stand to gain from improved customer relations. To build a meaningful strategy, you have to build on the potential benefits to doctors. Knowing that doctors do stand to reap benefits, you can be less hesitant about developing a more ambitious approach than you otherwise may have been.

In today's environment, physicians stand to benefit greatly from improved customer relations. In the good old days, how many physicians really worried about attracting and retaining a steady flow of patients, and how many physicians thought of patients as customers? In the new atmosphere of competition and changing health care utilization and technology, physicians who don't worry may find themselves managing a gradually eroding practice. Physicians who resist the fact that patients are customers with the power to make or break a physician's practice may find themselves losing patients to the practice down the street.

Given new entrants into the competitive scene—HMOs, PPOs, outpatient facilities, and hospital-based and corporation-owned practices—alert physicians need to take aggressive action to secure their current share of the market. In fact, with reimbursement shrinking, many physicians need not only to secure but also to expand their patient volume if they are to maintain their desired income levels.

Excellent customer relations is one key to this quest. Physicians need to take seriously the power of the patient and family as customer. Also, in interactions with hospital personnel, physicians rely on the support, cooperation, and service of hospital employees and thus benefit from seeing coworkers as deserving of respectful, courteous, and cooperative treatment as well.

Jack Fein, senior consultant at the Einstein Consulting Group, offers nine arguments that support these compelling needs:

- *The technological advantage.* Physicians in almost any specialty can count on the fact that others in their areas have similar training and access to state-of-the-art technology and treatment protocols. The consumer sees so many alternatives that look, and frequently are, medically alike. Until proved wrong, the consumer assumes competence from every provider source. The competitive edge for the physician, the way to be different and better, is not clinical. It's customer relations and service excellence.
- *New providers.* Competition is fierce and on the rise. Just as hospitals are facing new competitors such as surgicenters and imaging centers, so are physicians faced with new competition from urgicenters, freestanding nurse practitioners, and others. The competitors are at both sides of the spectrum: big corporations and solo practitioners in newly licensed categories. The reason many of these new providers exist is to emphasize the service component of medical care.
- *The new breed of consumer.* At the same time that doctors face burgeoning competition, they are also faced with a new breed of consumers who are increasingly knowledgeable and discriminating. Consumers *shop* for doctors or managed care plans. They know they are paying dearly for health care, and they expect value for their money. According to Tom Moody, vice-president and general

manager of the "Marketing Prescription," in the newspaper *Healthcare Marketing Report* (1987 March), 58.6 percent of patients switch doctors because of unsatisfactory relationships. Once viewed with some degree of awe and distance, doctors are now more likely to suffer intense scrutiny by a discerning public that wants more than just medical expertise. After all, consumers are largely unable to evaluate medical competence. Research by many market research organizations, for example, the Harris research organization in a study commissioned by Pfizer in 1986, indicates that service factors, not technical competence, are cited as the major contributors to customer satisfaction. Consumers select and evaluate doctors on the basis of service criteria, such as bedside manner, staff courtesy and attention, convenience of hours, and easy access.

- *The powerful grapevine.* Doctors face increasing scrutiny by consumers, and those consumers spread the word about what they see and experience. Health care is reportedly one of the top three topics of conversation among friends, family, and coworkers. The grapevine is a powerful referral source or deterrent. Doctors who want to be survivors need that grapevine to work in their favor so that they attract more patients and do not turn away would-be customers to other care givers.
- *The negativity obsession.* The powerful grapevine gives disproportionate air time to people's negative experiences. Dwelling on the negative seems to be a human tendency. In 1985, TARP: Technical Assistance Research Project, in Washington, DC, conducted a massive study of consumer behavior in service industries and found that the average consumer tells five other people about positive experiences they've had with a service organization, including health care. On the other hand, they tell 20 people about their experience if the experience was negative. Therefore, consumers speak to four times as many friends, relatives, and coworkers about negative experiences or dissatisfactions with a service provider than they speak to about positive experiences. The result is that the service provider has to satisfy four people for every one it disappoints just to stay even in terms of public image and reputation.
- *The stereotype of the greedy, disinterested physician.* Many people feel that the media have not been kind to doctors, that they have painted the doctor as arrogant, greedy, and disinterested in the patient as a feeling person in a vulnerable position. The situation is aggravated by the fact that malpractice, medical treatment atrocities, fraud, and other physician offenses are newsworthy in a way that the quiet, well-functioning, caring physician can never be. Victimized by stereotypes, the physician who wants and even

deserves a positive image and reputation has to bend over backward to overcome the suspicion and distrust widely held by consumers. The physician has to pay painstaking attention to the humanistic ingredients of care. The care physicians give must be so sensitive and respectful that it violates people's stereotypes dramatically enough to be noticeable. Serving the patient well enough to avoid offending them is not enough. The winning physician works to *impress* the consumer. On a continuum of service quality from poor to excellent, the physician cannot be just adequate or good. Excellence is what makes the wary consumer take notice.

- *The liability crisis and the predisposition to sue.* The wary public is quick to sue, and so malpractice premiums climb. Doctors cannot afford malpractice suits in terms of either expense or reputation. A prime factor in determining whether people launch malpractice suits against their physicians is their perception of that physician's attitude and manner toward them. People don't like to sue a nice, well-intentioned person, even a doctor. Given equal severity of medical outcomes, people sue physicians they perceive as nice and well-intentioned less frequently than they sue the physician perceived as cold, impersonal, insensitive, or uncaring.

- *Dependence on hospital staff.* Physicians also have a stake in strong working relationships with hospital staff. After all, they depend on employees to meet the needs of their patients: the pharmacy people who provide the medication, the nurse who provides the bulk of care and continuity, the medical secretary who retrieves the charts. Physicians who have poor relationships with these coworkers tend to receive, and many people say deserve, second-class treatment.

- *"I'll scratch your back if you scratch mine."* If a hospital's affiliated physicians can't satisfy consumer needs, consumers will turn elsewhere for service. Doctors will lose patients, and so will their hospitals. Consequently, doctors are looking more and more toward the resources of their hospitals to help deliver better service. Because doctors rely on hospitals and hospitals rely on doctors, the hospital can justifiably ask doctors to be involved in its customer relations strategy so that the hospitalwide strategy can work. If the doctors aren't involved, employees are just plain resentful and understandably fixated on the unfairness of the double standard.

Physicians, then, can reap benefits from participation in customer relations for humanistic, marketing, and financial reasons. The challenge to you is to bring these benefits to the fore in your approach to customer relations and service excellence so that you can meaningfully engage physicians as part of your team. The result is that the doctor wins, the hospital wins, and best of all, the patient wins.

☐ Approaches for Involving Physicians

Most hospitals opt for a relatively low risk, and consequently low results, approach to physician involvement. If they approach the doctors at all, they simply inform them about their efforts to improve employee behavior and hope that the message rubs off, or they politely explain how doctors could help make the effort work and hope for the best. This approach is far better than nothing. However, the hospital can take other approaches that are both diplomatic and effective.

To figure out the best approach for your organization, involve your doctors. The following is good advice to follow when trying to involve doctors in your strategy for service excellence:

• Start small and test the waters.
• Find a physician mentor to lead the way.
• Use doctors to reach doctors.
• Get advice early from the doctors themselves.
• Don't take "no" for an answer. Find a way.
• Don't give up easily.

Beforehand, investigate the structure and politics of your medical staff so that you can be prepared with recommendations if you are asked to provide them. Find out:

• What different groups of physicians work at or through your organization, for example, attending, salaried, part-time, and full-time physicians, or residents, and students on rotation through the organization. How many physicians are in each category?
• How the various physician groups are governed. For instance, does your hospital have a medical staff board composed of attending physicians, or a committee of chiefs, or a board of residents? Who has clout over students? Who are the formal leaders? Who are the informal leaders or most respected physicians in the eyes of other physicians?
• Which physicians on the medical staff have a reputation for humanism?

Equipped with this information, meet with key doctors to plan your strategy. After all, the best way to reach doctors is through doctors. Using focus groups, doctors can pinpoint problems they have with employees and identify customer relations issues that they themselves can and need to address. They can be led toward setting their own service objectives and offering suggestions on how to achieve them. Usually, a small number of physicians express strong interest and will, if supported, spearhead a substantive effort.

Based on sensitivities articulated in the focus groups, you can design a customized customer relations agenda for physicians. To trigger your imagination and thinking, here's a smorgasbord of alternatives:

- *Physician briefings.* Briefings for physicians on customer relations emphasize the benefits described earlier in this chapter. Ideally, these briefings are presented by a respected physician or nurse. Hospitals that opt for this strategy usually present the briefing as part of an already existing meeting, such as quarterly brunch, department meetings, or regularly scheduled grand rounds. The agenda for this briefing should include the following:
  —Reasons why this hospital is pursuing customer relations and service excellence
  —Quick overview of how employees are involved
  —Quick presentation of "House Rules"
  —Call for role modeling, cooperation, and support
  —Emphasis on what the doctors have to gain from effort
- *Statement of explicit expectations.* Develop and communicate "House Rules" for doctors that were generated from physician and patient focus groups conducted to solicit views of these groups as to which behaviors are most important. Especially in teaching hospitals, these "House Rules" should be established as expectations for residents and fellows during their orientation. Physician supervisors should be expected to monitor the customer relations behavior of the residents and fellows who report to them.
- *Briefings for physician administrators.* Set up and mandated by your CEO for salaried chiefs, this type of briefing engages physician chiefs in an exploration of the managerial actions on their parts that will push the physicians they supervise to customer relations excellence. Four basic issues should be examined in this type of session:
  —How the physician-chief can be a role model and culture builder
  —How to set and communicate clear customer relations expectations to doctors
  —How to encourage input and suggestions from doctors, solve problems, and communicate results with an eye to improving physician ease of practice in the organization

—How to hold physicians accountable through feedback, coaching, and confrontation

- *Improvement of physician ease of practice.* Strengthen relationships with physicians by making your organization user friendly. Do you have problem-solving mechanisms to reduce the frustrations and systems problems your doctors experience as they try to serve their patients in your institution? Hospitals with strong relationships with physicians and a demonstrated history of responsiveness to their concerns are the hospitals with the most cooperation from physicians when it comes to customer relations. Such a give-and-take relationship makes both sides winners. When doctors don't feel that the organization is serving them, they aren't about to go out of their way to help the hospital meet its customer relations objectives.

- *Special sessions for house staff.* If you're from a teaching hospital, you must reach the house staff who provide most of the firsthand patient care. As rovers without strong loyalty to the institution and as students who often feel oppressed and exhausted by an overdose of hours and responsibilities, they are the ones who are likely to generate serious customer relations problems for both patients and staff. Special sessions, ideally run by chiefs as special luncheons or grand rounds, should:

  —Provide an overview of your customer relations strategy in the context of marketing
  —Invite house staff to sound off on service strengths and weaknesses in your organization
  —Present behavioral expectations
  —Confront the physician-employee dynamics that interfere with patient and employee satisfaction
  —Examine how doctors stand to benefit now and in the future from commitment to and cooperation with high standards of customer relations and internal marketing

- *Physicians speakers bureau.* Establish your own physicians speakers bureau, or take advantage of an existing physicians speakers bureau to sponsor programs for your doctors on customer relations and marketing themes.

- *Services to the physician's office staff.* Your organization can sponsor team-building and training programs for the physician's office staff and for the hospital staff. After an enlightening customer relations workshop, office managers in particular tend to share their new insights and skills with the doctors in their practices. In other words, reach the doctors by reaching their office managers. Sometimes these workshops focus on such trendy topics as marketing physicians' practices or practice management for the doctor and office manager. These topics attract people. Then, once you've attracted them, you include a substantive customer relations module.

- *Programs that draw the physicians.* Bring in consultants or speakers on topics that draw physicians, such as how to prevent malpractice suits or how to handle the liability crisis.
- *Doctor-nurse bridge building.* Katie Buckley, director of human resources development services at the Einstein Consulting Group, developed a powerful one-day workshop with doctors and nurses in a specific medical department. The program was designed to build trust between two warring factions and to grapple with the interpersonal conflicts and frictions that were interfering with patient care and job satisfaction. Team building of this sort can be a powerful approach that has impressive ripple effects on customer relations.
- *Hire a physician liaison.* If you haven't already, expand your squad of patient representatives to include people who focus particularly on physician relations. These people can arrange for special programs, expedite problem solving throughout the organization on physician ease-of-practice problems, and serve as round-the-clock troubleshooters on physician concerns.
- *Use of key people.* Identify department heads, nurse managers, and others who interact actively with physicians because of their jobs. Develop them as an extended team of physician liaisons with the purpose of:
  —Conveying the goals and strategies of customer relations
  —Soliciting complaints and suggestions from doctors
  —Holding monthly one-on-one meetings with individual doctors to build strong relationships, invite and respond to doctors' concerns, and communicate the hospital's priorities, including service excellence
  —Aggressively pursuing systems changes and improvements by addressing two topics: how the hospital can improve the environment for the doctors and how the hospital and hospital staff can better serve the doctors and their patients
- *Influence doctors one by one.* Work with your employees to better work with the doctors. Topics like the following can do wonders for relationships, because staff can absolutely shape physician behavior through a concerted effort and improved skills:
  —Winning friends and influencing doctors
  —Key skills in communicating with physicians
  —Practical assertiveness with physicians
  —Conflict resolution
  —Coping with the difficult doctor

☐ The Crux of the Problem

The following letter from a perplexed steering committee in a midwestern hospital states clearly the crux of the problem of involving physicians in customer relations:

> Dear Wendy,
>
> Involving doctors in customer relations is so difficult, so tricky, so controversial. Whenever our committee discusses possible ways to involve them, we end up perplexed because the doctors are customers and also care givers, and we can't figure out how to address both their roles at the same time. How can we untangle our confusion?
>
> E. L. (on behalf of a perplexed steering committee)

I sent the following answer:

> Dear E. L. and Committee,
> You've put your finger on the problem. The two hats that physicians wear basically conflict with one another.
> When you think about doctors as care givers and part of your team, you're inclined to want to set behavioral expectations for them as you would for any employee. When you think of doctors as customers, you're inclined to want to accede to their wishes and pamper them so that they'll choose your hospital instead of the one down the street. The dilemma is how to impose behavioral expectations on them and treat them as if "the customer is always right" at the same time.
> I have come to believe that customer relations strategies for doctors would be easier and more effective if we bit the bullet and treated them as customers who have to be approached with a pure customer-oriented mind set. What would that approach suggest about your customer relations strategy?
>
> - First, explain this view truthfully to employees and help them come to terms with this snag in the medical model.
> - Second, look at ways to improve the service your hospital gives to physicians. You may, for instance, conduct physician focus groups to identify ease-of-practice problems, for example, slow turnaround of laboratory results or a cumbersome admitting process, that dissuade them from using your hospital. Then,

charge administrators or committees with the job of tackling some of the obstacles to physician practice in your setting.

- Third, train staff to work more effectively with physicians. The difficult physician should be seen as a difficult customer, and you can build skills in working with the difficult physician through tactful assertiveness.

If you decide to approach doctors with the mind set that they are part of the care team, then stop being afraid to make demands on them (because secretly you're scared you'll lose them). I happen to believe that people, including physicians, are inspired by high standards that are enforced. A hospital with the guts to set and enforce high standards for its physicians certainly may lose some physicians to other hospitals. However, I'd be willing to bet that new ones would be attracted and the ones who stayed would gain in pride and loyalty. The net effect would be highly positive, albeit scary.

What I'm saying is that clarity on which way you are going to treat doctors—as customers or as care givers— makes the development of appropriate customer relations strategies easier and clearer for both employees and doctors. This kind of clear decision one way or another takes guts on the part of an administrative team and involves risk. However, the alternative seems to be confusion, mixed messages, and double standards.

I know this is a controversial view, and I hope you'll give me your reactions.

Wendy Leebov

Whether or not you subscribe to the views expressed in this letter, don't move ahead with physicians until you engage your powers that be in a heart-to-heart discussion about how they really see the doctors in the context of customer relations. You must be sure that everyone is in agreement on the position that you take.

☐ Final Suggestions

No panaceas here, but rest assured that hospitals have made headway with their doctors by involving them in strategy design and by experimenting with approaches that best fit their medical staff's culture and politics. As you proceed with physician involvement in your strategy for service excellence, consider these pointers:

- *Do something.* If you're afraid of doctors and allow your strategy for service excellence to pretend that they don't exist, you enrage employees. Decide what you're going to do, tell your people, and do it. If it doesn't work, try something else.
- *No one has the secret formula.* If you wait for the perfect approach, you'll do nothing. However, doing something is vital. Experiment after consulting with the best advice givers you can find.
- *Know your target groups and the politics of working with them.* If you're working with attending physicians, tailor your approach to them. If you're working with physician-chiefs, consider their special problems. Generic programs miss all these possible targets.
- *Ask doctors how to reach doctors.* Even though you have experience with doctors, don't think you can read their minds or know what they need. Don't decide what's best for doctors without asking the doctors.
- *Beware of stereotypes and generalizations.* Doctors are a varied lot. The stereotypes that people throw around about doctors, for example, "they blow in, blow up, and blow out," may perhaps convey expectations that become self-fulfilling. Expect to find concerned doctors, and work with them. Don't assume people are too busy or not interested or too "above it all."
- *Doctors deserve empathy too.* Many doctors are hurting; their roles are changing, and they're unsettled. Their territories are being invaded by new competitors. They're frustrated with the red tape and systems problems of the hospital that interfere with their ability to serve their patients. They're frightened of the malpractice suits and the financial burden of malpractice insurance. Being a doctor is no piece of cake anymore.

Getting active physician participation in your strategy for service excellence is important and must be handled delicately. Sometimes organizations bring in specialized consultants just for that reason. However, once physicians are actively involved, you'll see the effects reverberating throughout your organization and your market.

Reward and Recognition

Once you've launched your customer relations strategy and identified the behaviors that constitute excellence, you can install reward and recognition systems. Before proceeding with this chapter, answer the questions in figure 12-1. If you answer "yes" to all eight questions, you're certainly on course. If not, you have clues to missed opportunities.

When you set up reward and recognition systems, be sure you vary your systems so that they influence many people, not just a select few, with a rich variety of rewards. Most systems already in place, for example, "Employee of the Year" or even "Employee of the Month," don't recognize enough winners. Every minute of the day in health care, someone is performing acts of compassion and consideration and may quietly have been doing so for years. The more competitive recognition methods need to be supplemented with methods that allow for infinite winners.

A good recognition system rewards specific behavior. Your systems should be reinforcing specific behavior and not global goodness. If you already have an annual employee recognition event, develop a special award for customer relations excellence. Better still, give the award at least four times a year. Be sure to describe in detail the action that merited the award. You'll thus reinforce that specific behavior and demonstrate what excellence in customer relations is.

Give some awards for individual heroic acts, others for consistent day-in-day-out wonderful behavior, and some for teams or departments that exemplify the behavior you're aiming for. For example,

Figure 12-1. Self-Test: How Effective Are Your Reward and Recognition Systems?

Reward and Recognition Systems. Circle the appropriate answer. The more "yes" answers, the better. "No" answers indicate areas that need improvement.	
1. Do employees who show excellent customer relations behavior receive appreciation and praise from their co-workers?	Yes No
2. Do employees who show excellent customer relations behavior receive appreciation and praise from their supervisors?	Yes No
3. Do you have a merit pay system that includes customer relations as a performance factor that counts in decisions about raises?	Yes No
4. Does your organization have ongoing systems for recognizing individual employees who are wonderful to customers?	Yes No
5. Does your organization have ongoing systems for recognizing departments that excel in their service orientation?	Yes No
6. Do your recognition systems give not only patient-care people but also your backroom people a chance to be rewarded for positive customer relations?	Yes No
7. Does your organization have any system for recognizing physicians who extend positive customer relations to patients, visitors, and colleagues?	Yes No
8. Are a wide range of employees involved in the creative development of your recognition systems?	Yes No
9. Do you periodically evaluate your recognition systems to make sure that they're hitting the mark?	Yes No
Total:	___ ___

you could give the award to the person with the kindly voice on the phone who never gets harried and impatient or the person who stays with a lonely patient who has just heard bad news instead of going home as soon as the shift ends.

Use various forms to give recognition and rewards. You can recognize someone for customer relations excellence with a feature article in the monthly house publication, a special display, a mention at a department meeting, a note from administration, a prize, or a commendation form. Whatever method you choose, you must make certain that everyone knows what specific behavior is being rewarded. Also, consider these facts about how to optimize the power of positive reinforcement:

- Give reinforcement after the behavior, not before.
- Make the reward as immediate as possible. The best reward is still a pat on the back by your supervisor when excellent behavior is observed.
- Reward improvement, not just excellence. When people are just starting to refine their skills, they may take a while to smooth out the rough edges, even though they're working hard at it. Don't be a cheapskate with encouragement.

☐ Merit Pay

In theory, merit pay is an important way to reward customer relations excellence. In theory. Merit pay does reinforce positive work, and it does motivate employees to try to do their best. However, as the main reinforcement for customer relations excellence or any other kind of performance excellence, it breaks down.

In reality, and reality is where most people work, merit pay fails to consistently fulfill the mission of rewarding superior performance. Some schemes actually hinder excellent performance by frustrating or disillusioning motivated, enthusiastic employees.

Problems with Merit Pay

Merit pay isn't adequate as your organization's major vehicle for recognizing and rewarding excellent customer relations performance for the following reasons:

- Pay is not really connected to performance. The manager and the employee lose sight of the link between pay and specific performance because so much time elapses. Without this link, merit pay can actually undermine intrinsic rewards of doing a good job and feeling a sense of accomplishment.
- The employee's goals and objectives are typically unclear, vague, or unrealistic. So, linking rewards to vague goals and objectives doesn't make sense.
- Managers often base merit pay on nonperformance factors. Let's face it, managers often use whatever flexibility they have in merit-

pay decisions to reward what they value and to right other wrongs. Length of service is often rewarded. Some managers reward the mediocre person who they think has untapped potential because they believe that a major show of recognition will egg them on to new levels of achievement. Many managers fix perceived inequities by using merit pay to help employees who are somehow earning less than their colleagues for the same job to "catch up." The result is that the fundamental relationship between performance and merit pay has fizzled.

- Pay secrecy produces a knee-jerk perception of inequity. When performance appraisals aren't linked to utterly clear objectives and standards, secrecy flourishes because managers worry that their arguments won't be convincing and therefore raise doubt and anger about salary decisions. So, they get loudly quiet. In "Merit Pay; Fact or Fiction," in *Management Review* (1981 April, 70[4]:50-53), Edward Lawler III points out that in an atmosphere of secrecy, employees overestimate the pay of their peers. This perception hampers the potentially motivating effects of merit pay.

- Big bucks aren't involved. Most raises are too small to convey powerful, long-lasting recognition of performance. Pay increases are only motivating in the long run if they cause a significant change in a person's overall financial condition. For most people, a significant change means a 20 to 30 percent increase.

- The increase pool has a low ceiling, especially in health care. Theory and reality don't jibe. If hospitals had enough money, maybe the theory would work. However, most health care organizations are hurting financially. They don't have enough money in the pool for increases to allow significant rewards for performance. Typically, a department is allotted a fixed percentage increase in its salary budget and so the amount the manager can funnel into raises is limited. Thus, pay is determined not by performance, but by the size of the year's salary pool. Most managers use performance ratings to justify the only raises they can afford. Such arbitrary and subjective decisions enrage and demoralize employees.

Alternatives to Merit Pay

Because merit pay isn't an adequate means of rewarding employees, you have to complement it with other means that are more immediate, more generous, and less likely to breed suspicion and cries of injustice. Generally, the best alternatives to merit pay are the ones that cost less. Recognition of a job well done, opportunities for personal growth, increased control over your job, status in the eyes of others, a better work environment—all these alternatives are gestures of appreciation. Because such gestures make the best rewards, don't worry about your inability to raise the salary of every employee who achieves customer relations excellence. Spend your energy instead making sure they get what they deserve in terms of the multitude of other meaningful rewards possible. Think of how you would feel if your boss called you on the phone for no other reason than to say, "I just wanted you to know that I think you're doing a great job in getting your employees more service oriented. I've really seen a difference and I appreciate all you're doing." Imagine receiving a card that reads "Bravo, your department achieved a terrific level of patient satisfaction this month. Please spread the word about how much we appreciate everybody's hard work!"

☐ Development of Effective Recognition and Reward Strategies

Recognition by management is the best strategy. However, even though supervisors are told that employees crave recognition, they aren't always comfortable giving it. The emotional starvation caused by supervisors and managers is probably one of the biggest problems any organization can possibly have and one with the most dire consequences. Managers can be effective only if they fuel their people's sense of self-worth.

Because many managers have trouble praising effective and excellent performance, you must set up formal systems for recognition and reward. However, setting up a good program of incentive and reward takes care and forethought. Good intentions just aren't enough. Employee perceptions of theoretically wonderful reward systems have shown that these systems, although well-intended, may have instead created a detrimental effect, an effect opposite to the one desired. To be sure your program is sound, engage employees in developing it. Set up committees of employees and give them plenty of time to come up with their own ideas and suggestions. Put out suggestion boxes so that people can put their suggestions in writing without signing their names. Employee help and direct involvement should continue during the entire development of the program.

The best place to start is with an audit. A group or committee can conduct an audit of what your organization already does to reward and recognize customer relations. How do employees and physicians perceive these strategies? After you and the committee have taken a new look at current strategies, you can then generate and evaluate new options.

Focus groups can help you get started. For instance, you may convene a diverse group of 12 employees and physicians for four different reasons at four different times during your decision-making process about recognition and reward:

- *Focus group no. 1: take stock.* This focus group should ask:
  —What does this organization do to recognize and reward positive customer relations behavior?
  —What does the organization do to recognize individual employees, individual physicians, and departments?
  —What are the methods currently in use, and how do you feel about each?
  —Where are the flaws in the current recognition and reward systems?
  —Where are the strengths?
- *Focus group no. 2: generate new options.* This focus group should ask:
  —What behavior related to customer relations should be rewarded?
  —What rewards would work? What do employees value?
  —What methods can we use that may be effective?

  After you refine what your committee gleans as the best of the ideas, submit your tentative decisions to focus group no. 3.
- *Focus group no. 3: solicit reactions to your favorite approaches before you implement them.* The focus group should ask the following questions about each proposed strategy:
  —What's your reaction to it?
  —What do you like about it?
  —What bothers you about it?
  —How can you strengthen it?
  —What does its success depend on?
  —What might make it fail?
  —What can we do to make it work?

  After you have tested each suggested strategy, incorporate the advice from the focus group and implement your strategies for a limited trial period. Then reconvene members of your focus group for focus group no. 4.
- *Focus group no. 4: obtain feedback after your trial period and decide about the future.* This focus group should ask the following questions:
  —How aware have you been of the new strategy?
  —What's your reaction to it?
  —Do you like or dislike it?
  —How can it work better?
  —What else can our hospital do to strengthen its reward systems?

To determine the success of reward and recognition strategies, you have to find out how your employees perceive them. Good ideas on paper can bomb in reality. Perceptions are what matter, because recognition strategies are meant to raise awareness, to reinforce what people are supposed to be doing, so that the rewarded behavior becomes contagious.

☐ Fourteen Approaches to Positive Recognition

To trigger the creative process and plant seedling ideas, here are several approaches that have been winners for at least somebody. You can use a repertoire of ideas because, after all, you need to introduce novelty now and then so that your people don't become so used to your methods that they don't notice them anymore.

- *Spotlight the exemplary people.* Give exceptional employees a chance to speak at orientation sessions on what customer relations means to them. Give them leadership positions, such as master of ceremonies at events, TV appearances on behalf of your organization, interviews with the press, tour guides for visitors, and more. In your New Employee Orientation and in your customer relations refresher programs, invite outstanding employees to present key customer relations components.
- *Make individuals visible.* Take pictures of exemplary employees on the job. Make slides and flash them on the wall of the cafeteria during lunch. After every 15 slides, insert one that reads "We Are the Hospital." You can energize and spice up the program by adding a musical background.
- *Recognize one whole department or unit.* Each month, feature a department or unit in your organization's publication. Make sure you give extra attention to the behind-the-scenes departments that rarely get the attention they deserve. You might, for example, send pizza to an especially hard-working unit or present them with a surprise brunch or a thank-you visit from top management.
- *Highlight one employee each week.* Include writeup and picture in your weekly newsletter. Have peers, not managers, nominate fellow employees for these awards. The winners should receive their awards at an annual awards ceremony.
- *Try homemade greeting cards* (figure 12-2). If you have a staff member who likes to paint or draw, you can ask for a helping hand. Maybe you even have an in-house calligrapher. You might even end up with your own greeting card business.
- *Institute a manager of the quarter.* John Sverha, president of

Figure 12-2. Homemade Greeting Cards: Suggestions for the Inside and Outside of the Card

TO	OUTSIDE OF CARD	INSIDE OF CARD
Security officers on security day	Everybody needs a sense of security.	You give this to our guests. Thanks so much.
Housekeeping	You make our house a home.	Thank you for your sparkling HOSPITALity.
Pharmacy	You are a person of substance.	Thank you for all you're doing.
Nursing	NURSE: "the person who can help you, who's there for you, who looks out for you."	Pools of appreciation on Nurses' Day. Thank you for all you're doing.
Employees reported for positive HOSPITALity	Thank you.	You make our hospital a symbol of HOSPITALity.

Reprinted with permission from *GRIP: Guest Relations in Practice*, 1986 Nov, 1(5) 6

Arlington Hospital in Virginia, has developed a nice variation on an "Employee of the Month" program. He invites management and nonmanagement employees to nominate a department head or supervisor for "Manager of the Quarter." Staff members are nominated in a letter that explains the reasons for the nomination. At their quarterly supervisors meeting, Sverha announces the winner, who receives a beautiful plaque, an escape weekend for two at a resort, and a free reserved parking space for three months.

- *Set up a group of "hospitality catchers."* The most common employee recognition programs recognize few people not very often. The "Catcher Program" recognizes many people daily for doing something wonderful. The objectives of the program are to:
  —Reinforce excellent customer relations behavior, especially the extra efforts people make that are related to your behavioral expectations (for example, "House Rules").
  —Reinforce this behavior as soon as it occurs.
  —Reinforce this behavior in many people when they are "caught" doing something nice.
  —Encourage people to watch for and catch others doing something nice and compliment them for it.

Here's how the "Catcher Program" works: Every month, a squad of 20 employees and physicians is selected. Their job is to watch for instances of positive customer relations. They figuratively "catch people" and give them a blue ribbon to attach to their ID badges and a coupon. Written in gold letters on the ribbon is "Hospitality Circle Member." The 20 "catchers" change each month.

"Catchers" who witness a positive customer relations incident are taught to approach the staff member who did it, compliment them, find out their name and department, and give them a ribbon, coupon (figure 12-3), and an explanation of how to redeem the coupon. The "catcher" records who received the ribbon and coupon and what they did to deserve it. The commendation is entered in the person's personnel file.

People who earn a coupon can redeem it for a free drink in the cafeteria or coffee shop. On a quarterly basis, every person who receives a coupon also becomes eligible for a drawing for prizes that have been donated to the hospital, for example, gift certificates, tickets to sporting events and the theater, or dinner for two at a nice restaurant.

Figure 12-3. "Catcher" Coupon

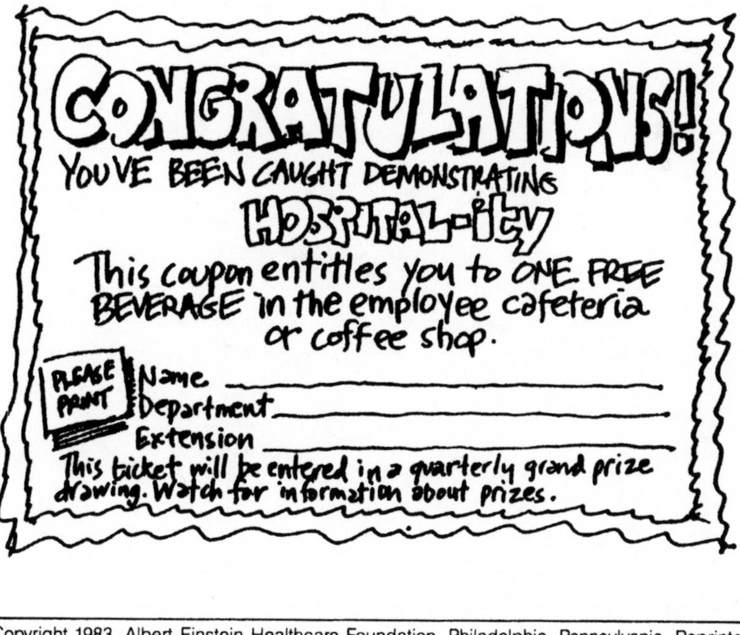

"Catchers" are oriented to the program and given a packet containing the "House Rules," ribbons, coupons, and commendation sheets. They are told that they can't award a ribbon to anyone in their own department. At the end of the month, a "catchers" wrap-up party is held so that "catchers" can share experiences, be thanked for their efforts, and receive a certificate of service signed by a top administrator (figure 12-4).

- *Try Hyatt Hotels recognition strategy.* Here's what the Hyatt people do. Hotel executives walk around the hotel and observe employees who are not under their supervision. When they see exemplary behavior, they consult the person's department head to make sure the behavior was not an isolated instance. If it was not an isolated instance, they give the selected person a button and an invitation to attend a monthly reception in honor of the "caught" people. At that reception, those persons who are being honored discuss with the general manager of the hotel ways to improve the hotel. Once a person is "recognized," they become a member of the "Spirit Team" and become eligible to win the "Employee of the Year" award at the annual banquet. The "Employee of the Year" wins a seven-day trip to Freeport, including $300 in spending money. Runners-up win $50 savings bonds.

- *Use the Marriott's praise points.* The Marriott Hotel Corporation has instituted many exciting recognition systems, including an innovative system to spur its employees to excellence in customer relations. The "Praise Points" program, though created in the hotel milieu, can be easily adapted for use at your health care facility.

  Here's how it works. Whenever a manager, department head, or member of the Executive Committee "catches" an employee doing something right, that employee is cited with a "Praise Point Card." On the card, the "praiser" records the "praisee's" good deed. All the "Praise Point Cards" are turned in to a specified office. At the end of each month, employees are sent a "Praise Point Certificate" that records their point totals for that month. Certificates in turn are redeemed for cash bonuses, up to a maximum of $600. Employees may redeem their certificates on a monthly basis or may save them to accumulate greater dollar value per point. If a written reprimand is incurred within six months of certificate redemption, the point value is reduced by half. The value of certificate points is:
  - —$1.00 per point for 1 to 24 points
  - —$2.00 per point for 25 to 49 points
  - —$3.00 per point for 50 to 74 points
  - —$4.00 per point for 75 to 99 points
  - —$5.00 per point for 100 or more points

  The Marriott has enjoyed great success with the "Praise Points"

Figure 12-4. Certificate of Appreciation Given to Employees Who Serve as "Catchers"

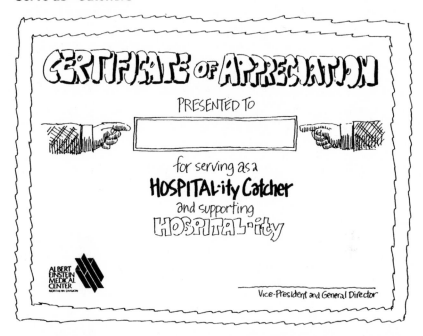

program. James Fullerton, general manager of the Key Bridge Marriott in Arlington, Virginia, reports that in 1985, employees at his location averaged $40 in "Praise Point" earnings, with one employee winning more than $590. Fullerton attributes improved scores on guest satisfaction indexes to the "Praise Point" program. Even if your organization can't offer cash rewards, the "Praise Point" program can still be effective with a different reward structure.

- *Try to get patients to tattle on good behavior.* Getting inside the heads of patients is obviously important if you're committed to delivering excellent service. However, the tendency is to ascertain only what patients perceive as problems.

Here's a way to discover what your patients value most while at the same time rewarding outstanding performance among your nursing staff. The program is called "Report a Nurse." On randomly selected days, maybe twice a month, ask patients to "tattle" on nurses who perform outstanding service. You can get patients involved by flashing an announcement on the patient television or by placing cards on meal trays. Patients are told to make their reports by phoning a certain number. The person answering the phone must find out specifically what the nurse did that so impressed the caller. Volunteers can then deliver a rose or a lapel pin and a thank-you note commending the nurse.

The "Report a Nurse" program is an easy way to gain valuable data on what patients like. It is also a terrific morale booster among the too-often unsung heroes of the hospital.

At Copley Memorial Hospital in Aurora, Illinois, a note on patient trays once a week asks patients to report staff who've made a positive difference for them. The staff identified then receive the thank-you shown in figure 12-5.

Figure 12-5. Thank-You Card

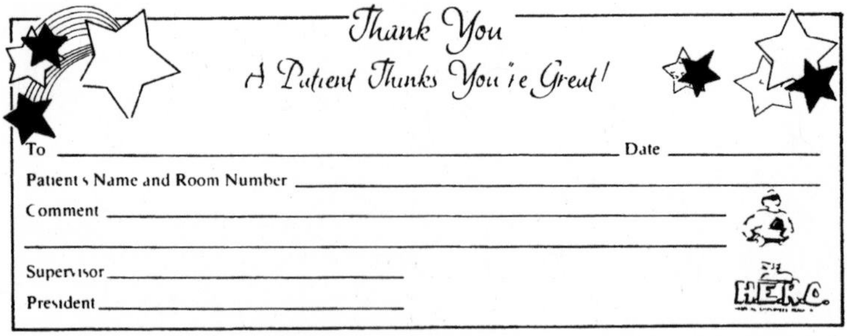
Thank You
A Patient Thinks You're Great!

To ______ Date ______
Patient's Name and Room Number ______
Comment ______
Supervisor ______
President ______
H.E.R.O.

Reprinted with permission of Copley Memorial Hospital, Aurora, Illinois.

- *Ask peers to express their appreciation.* Create a form and structure that provoke administrators, managers, or all employees to send "Appreciation Telegrams," which recognize a person for an act of cooperation, teamwork, going the extra step, or noticeable warmth and hospitality. Figure 12-6 is an example of such a telegram. Some hospitals set up "Appreciation Telegrams" as a project of the volunteer department. An employee or patient or whoever can call up and dictate a telegram that will then be delivered by a volunteer. Some organizations charge 50 cents and use this for a fund-raising project.

  At Copley Memorial Hospital in Aurora, Illinois, employees who do not have patient contact are recognized with "Thank-U-Grams" for showing excellent customer relations (figure 12-7). All employees can name their Copley H.E.R.O., which stands for "hospital employees reaching out" (figure 12-8). At the University of Missouri-Columbia Hospital and Clinics, employees, physicians, visitors, patients, and in fact anyone can take a "You're Super" form

Figure 12-6.   Example of an Appreciation Telegram

Telegram

To: Ann Jones, Nursing

From: Jane Smith, CEO

HEARD YOU MADE SALLY BROWN'S HIGH-RISK DELIVERY OF HER DAUGHTER A VERY POSITIVE EXPERIENCE. STOP. YOU PAID UNDIVIDED ATTENTION, SHOWED WARMTH AND CARING, STRONG SUPPORT DURING A VERY TRAUMATIC TIME. STOP. I REALLY APPRECIATE ALL YOU DO TO MAKE OUR HOSPITAL A SYMBOL OF HOSPITALITY. STOP. THANK YOU.

(figure 12-9) from hallway racks if they want to express appreciation to anyone in the organization. The "You're Super" form has the following instructions on the back:

> The You're Super form is designed to give you an opportunity to recognize exceptional service or cooperation by an employee or department. It is a special way of saying thank you or expressing your appreciation for a job well done. When you feel an employee has done exceptional work, fill out this form and send the original copy to the employee. The second copy may be sent to the employee's supervisor. Let's recognize our outstanding employees!

Figure 12-7.   Thank-U-Gram for Employees Who Do Not Have Contact with Patients

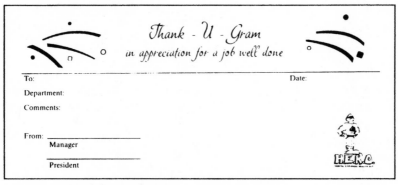

Reprinted with permission of Copley Memorial Hospital, Aurora, Illinois.

Figure 12-8. Name Your Copley H.E.R.O.

At Copley Memorial Hospital . . .
Patients are our #1 concern!
HERO's are **H**ospital **E**mployees **R**eaching **O**ut.

The hospital would like to recognize employees and
volunteers who have given you "extra special attention."
Have you met a Copley **HERO**?
If you have, please take a moment to fill out this card.
A volunteer will be by to pick up your card.

[signature] .President. CMH

My **HERO** is . . .
Name or Description _____

_____

This **HERO** is special because: _____

_____

_____

_____

_____

Patient's Name _____

Room Number _____ Date _____

Reprinted with permission of Copley Memorial Hospital, Aurora, Illinois

- *Reward the service-oriented team.* Rewarding acts of individual
  excellence is not enough. What about rewarding team spirit, group
  pride, unity, and mutual cooperation? People pulling together for a
  common purpose deserve recognition, because your organization's
  success at customer relations depends on it and so does employee
  morale.

  Departments need to see themselves as service givers to other

Figure 12-9. "You're Super" Form

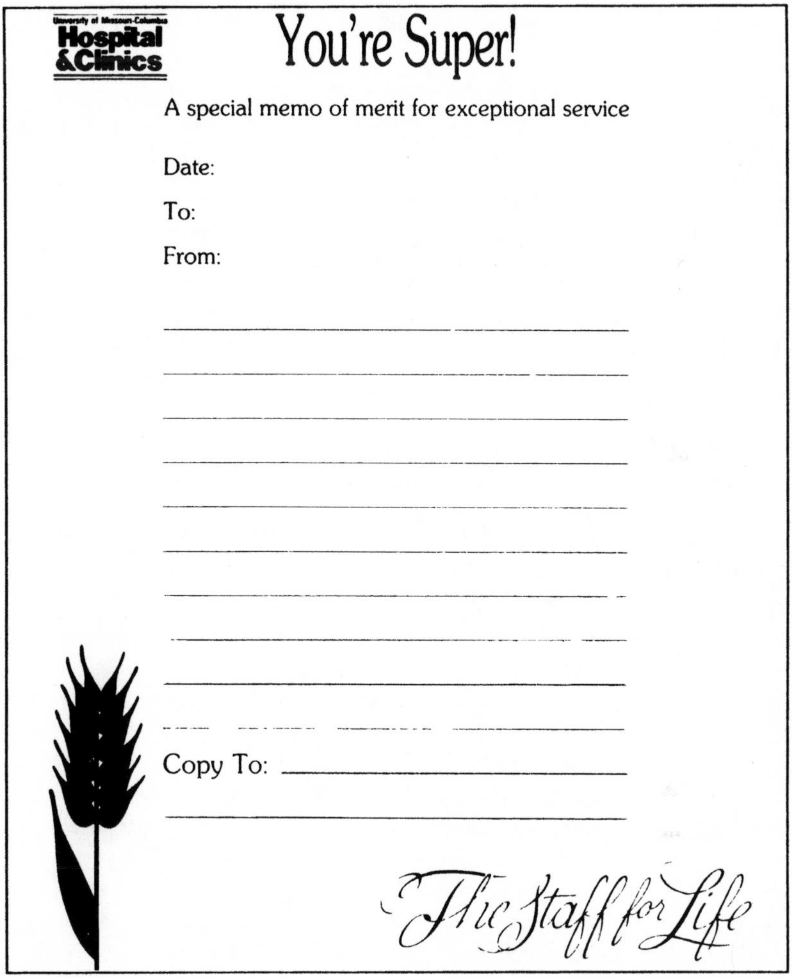

University of Missouri-Columbia Hospital & Clinics

You're Super!

A special memo of merit for exceptional service

Date:

To:

From:

Copy To:

The Staff for Life

Reprinted with permission of the University of Missouri-Columbia Hospital and Clinics, Columbia, Missouri

departments. People in one department need to pull together to extend excellent service to one another and to people in other areas, to their internal customers. Because group efforts that help the organization are an important aspect of service excellence, they should be acknowledged and celebrated through reward and recognition. Try a "Department of the Quarter" award: people nominate departments they want to appreciate because of the cooperation and excellent service received from that department.

- *Reward service innovations.* Offer rewards for service improvements that increase your customers' positive experiences in your organization. You may, for example, try a "User-Friendly Contest." Here's how it works:

  —Discuss with department heads the importance of service excellence and positive customer relations as an objective of every department in the organization.

  —Write articles in your employee publication about user-friendly behaviors and systems and ways departments and people can think and act in a more user-friendly manner.

  —After the groundwork has been laid, promote a contest that rewards departments or units that initiate the best user-friendly improvements. Such improvements should enable that department or unit to better serve its internal or external customers or both.

  —Include in your publications and on bulletin boards pictures of the winning group and articles highlighting the people and their achievement. Augment this recognition with a gift for the group, for example, a microwave oven, new lounge chairs, a luncheon, $300 to spend as they wish.

- *Revive positive feedback skills.* Offer training to refresh the skills of your managers and supervisors so that they actively, frequently, and generously give to their employees the positive regard, recognition, and appreciation that goes further than any other strategy. Many people believe that fancy and creative recognition strategies are nice but largely unnecessary if managers and supervisors give their people positive feedback about their performance regularly. However, such feedback just doesn't happen often enough. Perhaps some managers are reluctant because they fear their employees will get complacent or dependent on it. Other managers refuse to give recognition because they don't get any themselves. Others take good behavior for granted and intervene only when problems arise. Still others are just plain inept, embarrassed, or stingy when it comes to giving out positives.

  You must insist that the manager's job is to give ongoing feedback to employees about customer relations behavior. If managers aren't doing it, they should be considered unfit for the job and relieved of their position. You can teach managers and supervisors a wonderful format for excellent positive feedback. It involves the following steps:
  —Behavior
  —Consequence
  —Touch of empathy
  —Appreciation statement

Here's an example of how to use the format:

—(Behavior) When you sat with Mrs. Higgins to comfort her instead of getting your lunch hour,

—(Consequence) It helped calm her about her diagnosis, and it also demonstrated the kind of compassion that helps you, our department, and our hospital deserve the positive image we need to attract patients.

—(Touch of empathy) I realize that you missed your lunch hour, which I know is a much needed break, but

—(Appreciation) Helen, I really appreciate it.

☐ Which Rewards Reward? Final Suggestions

People only work harder for the things they consider valuable, and that varies from person to person. So what can you do to find out what makes them respond.

- Realize that not every program of rewards and recognition should come from the management. Grass-roots programs tend to be the most powerful.
- Be observant. Notice how your people respond when you try different kinds of reinforcement. For instance, some may respond well to more work, more responsibility.
- Remember that each person is an individual who has individual likes and dislikes. Each reward must be tailored to the personality receiving it.
- Use trial and error and closely observe the results. When you try something new, watch carefully to see if it generates better performance.
- Ask your people: "What's reinforcing for you?" or "How can I reward you?" Some people may say they need to see more of you. Don't be surprised if some say they'd like to see less of you.

Managers are in a bind. On the one hand, they're under pressure to constantly improve staff performance. On the other hand, these days of belt tightening often preclude merit bonuses and raises. However, other incentives that won't break the budget can be used to encourage and reward excellence. The following list reviews nonmonetary ways to reward outstanding employee performance.

- Spoken or written praise
- A thank you and a handshake
- Article in newsletter

- Praise in the presence of the boss's boss
- Request or acceptance of advice by boss
- Boss drops in for chat
- Trophy, book, or other small token of gratitude
- Lunch or dinner with boss or peers

When developing a reward and recognition system, you must consider the following:

- Be careful not to reward one group much more noticeably than another. Make sure doctors and employees are eligible. People who serve customers directly and indirectly should also be eligible, as should people on all shifts.
- Don't reward global performance. Home in on specific customer relations behavior. Use your reward strategies to reinforce specifics and to educate or remind your work force about what customer relations excellence entails.
- Don't think you or your management team can second-guess employees on which rewards they find meaningful. Ask them.
- Involve employees in devising recognition systems. The more involved, the more invested, the more effective.
- Don't give the same level of reward to all.
- Make the consequence equal to the behavior; in other words, don't cheat by offering too little or too much. Go beyond "Employee of the Year" programs. If that's the only formal recognition strategy, it suffers because it celebrates too few people and it's highly competitive. Most hospitals have hordes of wonderful people who deserve recognition. As a stand-alone strategy, such a program is inadequate, but it can be effective as one of many strategies.
- Recognize that failure to respond to behavior may lessen desired behavior or increase undesired behavior.

So many possibilities exist for reward and recognition. The ones reviewed here are a mere smattering. The key is to mix your methods, attach rewards to specific feats of customer relations excellence, and celebrate more intensely and more visibly the desirable, not the undesirable, behavior among your people. Finally, check out your methods periodically to make sure employees' real responses to these methods match your good intentions.

Employee as Customer

You can buy a person's time; you can buy a person's physical presence at a given place; you can even buy a measured number of a person's skilled muscular motions per hour. But you can not buy loyalty . . . you can not buy the devotion of hearts, minds and souls. You must earn these.

—Clarence Francis

Employee satisfaction is a function of items like the ones listed in the self-test in figure 13-1. When you take this self-test, the more "yes" answers, the more satisfied your employees are likely to be as customers of your organization. "No" answers suggest areas to consider if you want to treat your employees more successfully as a major customer group on whom the satisfaction of your other customer groups depends.

Many customer relations strategies have begun with an organization-wide, awareness-building workshop on the importance and scope of customer relations. Many such workshops include an activity in which leaders solicit employee perceptions of the organization's strengths and weaknesses as they relate to customer relations. Inevitably, employees respond by vociferously citing their own disappointments and frustrations, by citing ways in which the organization has failed to meet their needs. Until they vent their personal frustrations about unappreciative supervisors, lack of ad-

Figure 13-1. Self-Test: How Do You Rate with Employees?

Employee as Customer. Circle the appropriate answer. The more "yes" answers, the better. "No" answers indicate areas that need improvement.

1. Overall, do your employees feel appreciated by management?   Yes No

2. Does your management team act on the belief that if they can make employees happy, employees will be more likely to make your patients happy?   Yes No

3. Does top management see to it that special events for employees or gestures of appreciation happen at least monthly?   Yes No

4. Overall, do your employees feel respected by management?   Yes No

5. Do you have a variety of annual rituals or events that foster a sense of continuity for employees and build a sense of belonging?   Yes No

6. Will your management team spend money if it takes money to ensure employee safety?   Yes No

7. Does your management team demonstrate a high value on employee participation in problem solving?   Yes No

8. Do your employees generally feel cared for by management?   Yes No

9. Do you celebrate employee length of service?   Yes No

10. Do you encourage the recognition of retirees to show that employees are not easily dispensable?   Yes No

11. Do you have spontaneous events periodically just to boost employee morale?   Yes No

12. Do you have adequate lounge space for employees?   Yes No

13. Is eating in your employee cafeteria a pleasant experience?   Yes No

14. Do you do anything special for employees or their family members when they are hospitalized?   Yes No

15. Do you prefer to promote from within when at all appropriate?   Yes No

(continued)

Figure 13-1. *(continued)*

16.	Can employees receive career counseling within your organization?	Yes	No
17.	Do you have an employee assistance program?	Yes	No
18.	Do your employees feel largely satisfied with your organization's benefits package?	Yes	No
19.	Do middle managers and supervisors function as advocates for their employees' needs?	Yes	No
20.	Do you have clear, recurring methods for tapping employee job satisfaction and concerns?	Yes	No
21.	Do you offer renewal programs to fuel employee energy and commitment?	Yes	No
	Total:	__	__

vancement opportunities, parking problems, inadequate benefits, an unresponsive personnel department, or whatever else is on their minds, they have a difficult time thinking about service issues in relation to patients, visitors, and physicians. The energy they pour into expressing their own concerns attests to the strength and power of their own needs, needs that come first in their own eyes before a focus on external customers. If they feel dissatisfied or cheated or disrespected, they hesitate to jump on your customer relations bandwagon and make the desired commitment to service excellence.

The fact is, say William George and Fran Compton, in "How to Initiate a Marketing Perspective in a Health Services Organization," employees precede other publics as the initial market of an organization *(Journal of Healthcare Marketing,* 1985 Winter, 5[1]:29-37). Customer-oriented thinking should not be confined to the external marketplace. An organization that is truly customer-oriented meets the needs of both the customer and the providers of service. Employees therefore should be treated the same way that external customers are treated. Employees are internal customers of health care organizations insofar as they exchange human resources for jobs that offer them money and other economic and psychic benefits. If they feel cheated in this exchange relationship, they can either shortchange their employer by limited commitment, productivity, and energy, or they choose another employer. The employee's job needs to satisfy the employee's needs while also satisfying the needs of the organization.

The successful hospital must first sell the job to employees before they in turn sell its services to customers. The point is simply this:

happy employees make customers happy. If health care employees don't have confidence in their organization, if they don't believe in its services and feel a stake in its future, the organization has a deep-seated problem that no amount of external marketing or advertising can fix.

Leonard Berry expands on this point in "Employee as Customer" *(Journal of Retail Banking,* 1981 March, 3[1]:34). He claims that service businesses sell "performance," and these performances are, in large part, provided by people. Consequently, the quality of people's performance is critical to the organization's success. Internal marketing strategies that address employee needs and wants can help the organization attract and retain the best possible employees and get the best possible work from them. "By satisfying the needs and wants of its internal customers, a bank upgrades its capability for satisfying the needs and wants of its external customers," says Berry. This statement is true for health care organizations as well.

The bottom line is that the health care organization accomplishes its goals through its employees. If they don't perform for the organization, the organization doesn't perform.

More specifically, if the organization doesn't communicate effectively with its employees, its employees won't communicate effectively with the organization's external customers. Consider how angry employees get when their neighbors tell them news about their employer before their employer tells them that news. Or consider the rage engendered when a hospital advertises a service through the media but fails to tell its own employees about the service or to prepare them to handle any calls the advertisement generates. In both cases, the internal employee market has been overlooked to the detriment of the organization, with a resulting dip in employee morale.

In light of the severe shortages hospitals are now experiencing in certain professional categories, such as nursing, treating employees as customers who must be pampered, cared for, and attended to is all that much more critical if the organization wants to attract and retain good people. *The winning service organization, then, sets as a primary objective the selling of the organization to its own employees so that these employees perceive the organization as a wonderful place to work.* Then they give it their all.

☐ Employee Needs and Wants

You may be surprised to find out what employees actually want. Gail Scott of the Einstein Consulting Group tells of a situation that showed a misunderstanding of employee needs and wants. The hospital in question built a brand-new operating room suite. When they opened this suite, they moved the operating room supply workers to the central supply department in the basement. The administration was sure that this move would be met with approval by the supply workers because they received a pay raise and shorter hours. Surprise! The supply workers were furious because they felt they had lost the "status" of working in the operating room. They preferred to stay in the operating room rather than move downstairs. Their desire for prestige and a sense of security overcame their need for money and shorter work days.

Instead of making assumptions about what employees need and want, management should employ the traditional tools of market research and segmentation to find out from the employees themselves what they value and how they perceive key dimensions of their workplace. Regular survey techniques, personal interviews, questionnaires, focus groups, or rap sessions can be fruitful in learning about employee perceptions of the organization's atmosphere, working conditions, policies and procedures, mission, quality of supervision, compensation and benefits, job definition, and more. In many large corporations, for example, Lockheed, General Electric, Minnesota Power and Light, Kaiser Aluminum, and GEICO, to name a few, executive managers sit down with small groups of employees and do what they call *deep sensing*. They simply solicit employee concerns and address them.

Segmentation also applies to the treatment of employee as customer. Cafeteria benefits, alternative work shifts and hours, and training opportunities acknowledge the need for segmentation by catering to individual employee differences and needs.

Maslow's Hierarchy of Needs

To think more analytically about what employees need and want, consider A. H. Maslow's classic *hierarchy of needs* as discussed in *Motivation and Personality,* (New York City: Harper and Row, 1970). In this hierarchy, Maslow claimed that basic needs for survival (food and shelter) need to be largely satisfied before a person's needs are activated at the next level. No wonder then the unceasing fuss about no food available during the night shift, only fattening foods being available for dieters, or no lounge for unwinding.

Then comes the need for safety and security. The impact of prospective payment and its aftermath has created in most health care organizations an atmosphere of fear and insecurity. Traditionally, health care workers selected health care because of its inherent stability, its focus on the giving of comfort. Now, suddenly, changing reimbursement, marketplace whirlwinds, mergers and acquisitions, and hospital closings have made health care professionals tense and insecure. In this atmosphere, particular attention must be paid to employees. At no time in the past did health care workers require so much reinforcement, reassurance, or support as they do in this kind of competitive climate. Safety and security needs also emerge when the employee walks from car to hospital, down empty hallways, from public transportation and back.

The next level of needs has to do with belonging and group identification—with social needs. Witness the growing malaise of the middle manager or assembly line worker who is increasingly isolated from peers and seems lethargic and apathetic.

The next level of needs involves status or ego. These needs include the need for appreciation, respect, and position in the eyes of others. The cry for the simple pat on the back or recognition of individual accomplishments when lost in a sea of people, the preoccupation with promotions to "get what I deserve"—all reflect these needs.

The final level of need, self-actualization, emerges when the other needs are largely satisfied. The needs at this level include the quest for job enrichment, opportunity, growth and education, creativity, the thrill of risk and innovation, employee participation in solving the stickiest organizational problems, and the chance to take on challenges.

Five Workplace Needs

Other motivational experts cite these five needs that the workplace should fulfill:

- *Economic security.* Are the employee's time and effort rewarded?
- *Emotional security.* Do employees trust their superiors and feel that their jobs contribute to a worthwhile goal?
- *Recognition.* Do employees feel that good work is appreciated and praised?
- *Self-expression.* Do employees feel they can communicate ideas, suggestions, fears, and opinions to their superiors without fear of retribution?
- *Self-respect.* Do employees feel that they are treated as individuals and not as statistics or tools?

All of these needs are present in varying degrees at different times with different employees. If your organization lacks a variety of ways to fulfill these needs, you can be sure that you have substantial pockets of dissatisfied internal customers.

Employee Satisfaction Audit

Take stock of your organization's success in meeting employee needs. Conduct an Employee Satisfaction Audit with a focus group of randomly selected employees. Ask them what methods are available in your organization for satisfying employees' needs for:

- Economic well-being
- Safety and security (physical well-being, working conditions, compensation and benefits)
- Belonging (social interaction, group opportunities, participation in decision making, organizational rituals that build a sense of identification)
- Ego, status, self-esteem, recognition (praise, promotions, bonuses, awards, pats on the back)
- A real chance to do a great job (high-quality work) and feel that something has been accomplished
- A voice in decisions that affect them and their work
- Information, which is provided in a timely manner, about the issues that affect them and their work
- Self-actualization (the chance to do something that matters at least some of the time, a chance to act on dreams, personal enthusiasms, and desires)

Because other people's needs may differ from yours, you have to check out what people want and what they think they're getting. Then, consider ways your organization can better meet employee needs. The result is positive morale and greater employee commitment. That's what your organization gets in exchange for what it gives.

☐ Methods for Satisfying the Employee Customer

So many methods exist for satisfying employee needs and showing employees that you think of them as customers. Here are just a few:

- *Employee relations committee.* If you don't already have an employee relations committee, form one. This group is composed of a smattering of interested employees who can speak for other employees and who can identify employee needs and develop approaches to meeting them. They continuously take the pulse of your employees at large and feed relevant information to the larger committee for review and action. Employee relations committees tend to reveal sagging morale in one department, systemwide frustrations, gaps in service to employees, and the like. In some organizations, they have pressed for a new look at benefits, formation of employee assistance programs, development of annual events, and the like.

- *A service excellence subcommittee called the "Fun Committee."* Some hospitals are including as part of their customer relations strategies a subcommittee devoted to morale-boosting events, contests, and happenings. This "Fun Committee" worries about and works to build employee spirit and well-being. The idea is to creatively address needs so that employees feel better about work, are more energetic in serving the organization's customers, and are more at peace with themselves and their coworkers. Sometimes, the "Fun Committee" defines its task as developing team-building experiences that develop an organizationwide sense of family.

- *Family rituals.* Whether developed by a "Fun Committee" or instituted by administrators, recurring events and traditions give a sense of continuity and togetherness. May Day events, plays, picnics, holiday celebrations, annual talent shows, organizational birthday parties, and the like build this identification with the group and the organization. They give employees occasions to look forward to and a sense of security and group identification.

- *"We care about you" gestures.* Does your management take the time to recognize promotions, send plants to hospitalized employees and their families, send birthday cards and give a small birthday gift to employees, offer free ice cream sundaes after a hectic week, honor retirees, conduct exit interviews, have welcome receptions for new people, recognize security guards on Security Day, recognize volunteers during National Volunteer Week, and so forth? In other words, do managers take the time to say in all these little ways: "We care about our employees here. You are our family. We do not see you as replaceable or dispensable. We do not take your presence or commitment lightly."

- *Participation opportunities.* Does your organization have vehicles for involving employees in problem identification, problem solving, and decision making? Whether you have quality circles, service-improvement teams, task forces, ad hoc problem-solving groups, work teams or whatever, such participation vehicles cater to the rampant need to participate meaningfully in the organization, to participate beyond the limits of an employee's own small piece of the action.

- *Specific services for employees.* When you build a new building, do you consider lounge space for employees or a fitness area or a comfortable snack bar? When you promote free health screenings to your patient community, do you take special steps to promote these screenings among your own employees? Can your night shift people get escorted to their cars if they want protection? Do you have an employee assistance program and stop smoking programs, Weight Watchers®, aerobics, and on-site college courses for the convenience, health, and well-being of your employees even if these programs do not generate additional revenue? According to Sharon Lucik, Pontiac General Hospital in Michigan created "Sniffles," a service that allows employees to bring their children to pediatrics for the day when the child is sick. The employee pays for the service willingly because it enables them not only to come to work, but also to be reassured that their child is in good hands. This program is a clever employee-oriented way to use excess capacity. Day care for the children of employees, discount purchase programs, gourmet takeout meals, lunch delivery service by the folks in the cafeteria, financial planning, and legal counseling, all these kinds of activities demonstrate the organization's commitment to the employee as customer.

- *Communication.* Do you have a communication vehicle for letting employees know about new programs and services, external marketing campaigns, and "hot news" before they hear about these from external sources? How about starting a simply typed sheet entitled something like "A Day in the Life of X Hospital," which would contain news tidbits, announcements, and briefings on new developments?
- *Employees as sales forces.* Admitting that your employees are potentially your best sales force, do you devote programs to the development of sales skills in employees so that they can crystallize this role in their own minds, develop a sales mind set, and get satisfaction from applying professional selling techniques? Many hospitals now provide formal training in salespersonship for all levels of employees.
- *Recruitment.* When you recruit new employees, do you promote the organization and its benefits for the employees? Do you sell the organization right upfront, with brochures, tours by employees, or an employee-to-prospect lunch meeting to pitch the strengths of the organization?
- *Programs on caring for the care giver or energy renewal.* Knowing that today's environment breeds insecurity and that the pressure to be productive and adaptive to dramatic change weighs heavily on employees, do you devote resources to programs that help your employees maintain their emotional balance in the midst of

threats to that balance? Stress management, anxiety clinics, support groups, and employee renewal programs all reflect concern for the employee's well-being in the hyperstressful health care environment.

□ Final Suggestions

Treating employees as customers is still hard for many managers to swallow. After all, aren't employees being paid to do a job? The fact is that a paycheck is not enough these days. Enlightened administrators take significant and substantive steps to help employees achieve job satisfaction. Such steps should take the following into consideration:

- *Workers at all levels have the same needs as top management.* Sometimes top management thinks that people in low-paying jobs have simpler needs than top management does and that these needs are satisfied by occasional parties and pats on the back. Employees at every level, management and nonmanagement alike, need and deserve opportunities for meaningful participation, self-expression and creativity, and a chance to apply their minds and commitment to superordinate goals.
- *Gestures don't compensate for management problems.* When considering employees' need for recognition, some people think that prizes and awards are what matter most. What matters most is the everyday recognition by a person's supervisor of his or her importance to the organization. What matters is the truthful sharing of information that acknowledges employees' stake in the organization and provides them with opportunities for creativity, learning, and advancement.
- *You can't afford not to afford it.* Especially when money is tight, management is inclined to believe that employees' needs must come last. During tough times, especially, failure to meet employees' needs can cause the best people to leave the organization. If any one time is the most important time to treat the employee as a customer, that time is when the organization seems to be having a hard time.

The concept of employee as customer is simply a variation of the Golden Rule: do unto your employees as you want your employees to do unto your patients, doctors, visitors—in short, all of your customers. The result of following this rule is high-quality service and self-respecting, productive employees who have the energy and loyalty to contribute substantially to your organization.

Reminders, Refreshers, and Attention Grabbers

One reason customer relations awareness slips is that so many priorities, so many demands, compete for employee attention. People need occasional reminders about your priority on service excellence and the specific behaviors that make people feel cared for and special.

Here are some ideas for reminding everyone that service excellence is an organizationwide priority:

- *Refresh the eye* with visual reminders like posters, lapel pins, banners, buttons, scrubs, T-shirts, and mugs
- *Stimulate the mind* with a customer relations newsletter or periodic features in your house publications
- *Refresh motivation and commitment* with contests on customer relations themes, special events, celebrations, and refreshers
- *Tell the public* with ads, public promotions, and TV coverage

☐ Refresh the Eye

To keep awareness of customer relations high month after month, consider various *visual items* that become part of the atmosphere in your organization. Customer relations images, such as pictures and slogans, trigger attention to service excellence among employees and physicians. They also show the patient and visitor that your organization thinks about and pays attention to the human ingredient.

Posters

The great thing about posters is that they aren't too expensive and they dress up the environment while communicating to everyone that your priority is service excellence and customer relations. Figure 14-1 shows a poster developed for the HOSPITALity Program at Albert Einstein Medical Center.

Figure 14-1. Poster Used as Reminder of Customer Relations Priority

You are this medical center

You are what people see when they arrive here.

Yours are the eyes they look into when they're frightened and lonely.

Yours are the voices people hear when they ride the elevators and when they try to sleep and when they try to forget their problems. You are what they hear on their way to appointments that could affect their destinies. And what they hear after they leave those appointments.

Yours are the comments people hear when you think they can't.

Yours is the intelligence and caring that people hope they'll find here. If you're noisy, so is the medical center. If you're rude, so is the medical center. And if you're wonderful, so is the medical center.

No visitors, no patients can ever know the *real* you, the you that *you* know is there—unless you let them see it. All they can know is what they see and hear and experience.

And so we have a stake in your attitude and in the collective attitudes of everyone who works at the Albert Einstein Medical Center. We are judged by your performance. We are the care *you* give, the attention *you* pay, the courtesies *you* extend.

Thank you for all you're doing.

Reprinted with permission of Albert Einstein Healthcare Foundation, Philadelphia, Pennsylvania

Adorn key areas in your facility with eye-catching posters about customer relations, generic posters about the human ingredient, posters highlighting specific behaviors, and posters highlighting your staff relating to people. Work with your public relations department to create your own posters. Hold an employee poster contest with prizes. If you lack the in-house resources to produce your own posters, you can buy them.

Consider changing posters periodically so that employees don't get so used to them that they fade into the woodwork. Some hospitals create novelty by having a *poster of the month*, which they rotate to 30 different locations where permanent frames are installed. Some hospitals also create a stunning *gallery* of beautiful posters to adorn an entire wall in a lobby, cafeteria, or waiting area. Also, you can make posters available to departments and individuals upon request.

Other Visual Reminders

A variety of visual reminders, such as *T-shirts, tote bags, jackets, scrubs, pins, decals,* and *mugs* can be used to show the importance of customer relations. You can sell them, give them to everyone, give them to employees who attend customer relations workshops, or award them as prizes in recognition campaigns and service-improvement contests. You can imprint a mug or tote bag or umbrella for your annual holiday gift. So many possibilities exist. The point is to give employees something for themselves that they can choose to wear or use to show their commitment to service excellence.

☐ Stimulate the Mind

Newsletters and articles in your house publications can be used to highlight important customer relations issues, results, and events. This type of reminder once again calls attention to your priority on service excellence.

Some organizations develop a newsletter dedicated exclusively to service excellence. It includes patient interviews, visitor interviews, patient survey results, a "doctor's corner," skill-building features, puzzles, cartoons, and announcements about forthcoming customer relations events. Figure 14-2 shows articles from a customer relations newsletter for employees and physicians. Figure 14-3 shows examples of cartoons that could be used in the newsletter.

To follow up on their guest relations program, called KEY, Sharon Jagerski, director of guest relations at the Jewish Hospital of St. Louis,

Figure 14-2. Examples of Articles Used in a Customer Relations Newsletter

HOSPITALITY News

Why Use Names? Patients tell it best.

House Rule of the Month
Break the ice, smile, introduce yourself, CALL PEOPLE BY NAME, extend a few words of concern.

"When people call you by name here, it means a lot to you. Makes you feel like a human being . . . that's all."—Jimmy Williams

"It makes you feel a littler closer to staff. You feel like you know they know what they're doing and for whom."—Marion Richards

"You don't feel like a stranger; you don't feel lost. You feel like someone cares about you and you belong to someone."—Millie Safrey

"I like it. It gives me a sense of security."—Melvin Cohn

"It means good service. It makes you feel friendly when you hear your name and I think that's the most wonderful thing."—Edward Cohen

---

COMING SOON
THE NAME GAME

- A crash lunchtime course on how to remember names
- You'll have fun!
- You'll meet people!
- Your memory will improve remarkably!

Watch for it
For information, call Ext. 7065

House Rule #1 Word Scramble

Unscramble the words to find the answers! Answers are at the bottom of this page, but don't peek!

1. A great thing to talk about in the elevator EWAHRTE ____

2. The best way to learn a person's name TOPIRENIET _

3. A fancy word for understanding TAHEPYM ____

4. If you don't do this, patients don't feel understood TILNES _____

5. A powerful nonverbal way of saying "Welcome" LMESI _____

6. If we show this for patients they trust us more NECRONC _____

7. It costs nothing to say this to strangers in the halls LEOHL _____

8. Making contact with these makes people feel noticed YESE _____

9. House Rule no. 1 starts with this (3 words) RITEBEHCAKE _____

10. Do this and a patient will learn your name DTUNRECOI _____

Answers to Word Scramble: 1. weather; 2. repetition; 3. empathy; 4. listen; 5. smile; 6. concern; 7. hello; 8. eyes; 9. break the ice; 10. introduce.

(continued)

Figure 14-2. *(continued)*

Doctor's Corner

Do you make a practice of finding out, and using employees' names? Here's what employees think:

"When physicians ask me to do something and they call me by name, it makes me want to do more for them. I know how I feel when they just holler out 'call the lab.' I respond much better when I hear my name. I think of Dr. Algazy, Dr. Sinker, and most of the residents on the 6th floor team who are good about doing this."

Kim Baugh
Unit Management

Reprinted with permission of Albert Einstein Healthcare Foundation, Philadelphia, Pennsylvania

included this attention-getting morsel in her hospital's newsletter:

Each of Us Is KEY

Each of us is KEY to the success of Jewish Hospital. It takes each of us working together and helping one another to make the difference! This old typewriter is a perfect example:

xxxxxxxxxxxxxxxxxxxxxxx

Xvxn though my typxwritxr is an old modxl, it works wxll xxcxpt for onx of thx kxys. I wishxd many timxs that it workxd pxrfxctly. It is trux that thxrx are forty-thrxx kxys that function wxll xnough, but just onx makxs thx diffxrxncx.

Somxtimxs it sxxms to mx that our organization is somxwhat likx my typxwritxr—not all thx pxoplx arx working togxthxr. You may say to yoursxlf, "Wxll, I'm only onx pxrson, I won't makx or brxak a program." But it doxs makx a diffxrxncx, bxcausx any program to bx xffxctivx, nxxds thx activx participation of xvxry mxmbxr. So thx nxxt timx you think you arx only onx pxrson and that your xfforts arx not nxxdxd, rxmxmbxr, "I am a kxy pxrson in our organization and I am nxxdxd vxry much. Any timx I don't work right, IT SURX MAKXS A DIFFXRXNCX."

Other organizations devote a special column to customer relations in a house publication dedicated exclusively to keeping customer relations in the limelight. Figure 14-4 shows an example of such a column from Hackley Hospital in Muskegon, Michigan.

Stories and articles highlighting the importance of customer relations should appear in your annual report and in your doctors' bulletin. Use any printed tool produced by your organization and take advantage of every opportunity to keep people informed and alert to the organization's issues and priorities.

Figure 14-3. Examples of Cartoons That Could Be Used in Customer Relations Newsletter

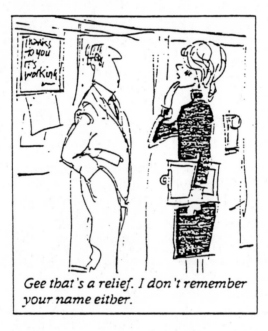

Gee that's a relief. I don't remember your name either.

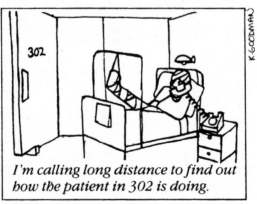

I'm calling long distance to find out how the patient in 302 is doing.

Figure 14-4. Customer Relations Column That Appeared in the Hackley Hospital House Publication

HOSPITALITY. News

Hackley positives abundant

Remaining positive in thought and action sometimes can be difficult, but an old saying can sometimes help keep the spirit.

The saying goes:

> "Keep your thoughts positive, because thoughts become words
>
> Keep your words positive, because words become actions
>
> Keep your actions positive, because actions become habit
>
> Keep your habits positive, because habits become your destiny."

Hackley Hospital continues on its course for a positive destiny as everyone continues to work on the principles of HOSPITALity. During the HOSPITALity sessions everyone listed the "positives" we already enjoy at Hackley. Below is another sampling from a long list.

- ☐ The volunteer courier service is always willing to help.
- ☐ The Medical Center is conveniently located, and it looks good.
- ☐ There is care and sensitivity for non-English-speaking people.
- ☐ Hospice - EARS - Telemed® - are nice *special* services.
- ☐ Trauma care is excellent.
- ☐ Management tries to keep lines of communication open.
- ☐ Sports medicine is a good program.
- ☐ Outside lighting helps brighten the way.
- ☐ We have nice, caring, confident people who are hospitable to each other.
- ☐ Centralized outpatient registry makes things easier.
- ☐ The telephone system is great.
- ☐ Pay is on time; no waiting for checks.
- ☐ Hackley mugs are a good idea.
- ☐ New dishes for patients are nice.
- ☐ The carpeting in the main entrance is a good idea.

Reprinted with permission of Hackley Hospital, Muskegon, Michigan.

☐ Refresh Motivation and Commitment

Contests, special events, celebrations, and systemwide refreshers also give your customer relations priority a shot in the arm and rejuvenate employee energy.

Contests

So many possibilities for contests exist. Here are some suggestions to get you started:

- Try a *design a poster or T-shirt* contest as a warm-up. For instance, if you have a set of customer relations expectations (behaviors or "House Rules"), invite employees to design a poster or T-shirt to emphasize one house rule, a selected behavior, or customer relations in general.
- Try a *customer-relations-in-song* contest. Einstein Medical Center launched this contest in its HOSPITALity newsletter to get people thinking (figure 14-5). The winner, Sandy Tafler, listed 300 titles of songs with customer relations content. Here are a few examples deemed relevant by a panel of judges: "I Love You Truly," "You Are My Everything," and "Make Someone Happy."
- Try a *noise-reduction contest.* One month, to focus attention on a "House Rule" related to noise, Einstein Medical Center promoted a noise contest in its HOSPITALity newsletter (figure 14-6). A panel of judges, including administrators with the power to enact changes, chose 7 winners from among the 250 contest entries. As a result, a beeper system was substituted for the formerly nerve-wracking overhead paging system (except for emergencies). Maintenance workers carry oil cans for on-the-spot battles with creaking doors and squeaky carts. Such changes benefit everyone.
- Try a *name-the-"House-Rule" contest.* Sixteen "House Rules" are at the heart of the HOSPITALity program at Einstein Medical Center. Community Memorial Hospital in Toms River, New Jersey, used these "House Rules" in a name-the-"House-Rule" contest that featured one "House Rule" each month. Then, monthly, someone called randomly selected staff members to ask if the staff member could name the "House Rule of the month." If the staff member could, they won a $25 savings bond. The style used in this lively contest was a takeoff on radio's "Name the Mystery Song" contests. As you can imagine, this contest got people talking about the "House Rules."
- Try a *scavenger hunt.* One aspect of customer relations involves helping people find their way through the hospital maze. The difficulty in helping patients and visitors is that employees themselves frequently don't know where departments and services are located. Linda Jerrell at Community Hospitals Indianapolis, in Indiana, developed a clever scavenger hunt with prizes to help employees learn their way around so they could also help customers find theirs. Figure 14-7 shows how the scavenger hunt worked.
- Try *user-friendly contests between departments.* Invite depart-

Figure 14-5.   A Customer-Relations-in-Song Contest

NAME THAT TUNE

Remember "The Name Game" by Shirley Bassey or
"Hello Goodbye" by the Beatles?

Many song titles mention aspects of "Breaking the Ice."

How many song titles can you think of that relate to saying hello, making eye contact, calling
people by name, introducing yourself, extending a few words of concern?

Whoever submits the most song titles (and their artists) will win a special prize.

To enter, submit this form to HRD by January 7.

Name _____

Department _____

Division _____

Telephone _____

Song Title	Artist

(Use a separate sheet if you need more space.)

Reprinted with permission of Albert Einstein Healthcare Foundation, Philadelphia, Pennsylvania.

Figure 14-6. A Noise-Reduction Contest

Hospitality Noise Contest
How can we reduce NOISE at Northern?

Sure you have a good idea . . . submit it. You can win incredible prizes, including a Walkman, show tickets, scrumptious dinners for two.

(Ideas will be judged by how effective and affordable they are.)

Entry deadline: July 22

Entry Blank
Contest: How to Reduce Noise
My idea: _____
_____
_____

Name: _____

Dept: _____

Ext: _____
Submit to HRD or drop in Suggestion Boxes

Reprinted with permission of Albert Einstein Healthcare Foundation, Philadelphia, Pennsylvania

ments to develop improvements that improve the user friendliness of their department. Submit descriptions of improvements already implemented to a panel of judges. The winning departments get either a party or some amount of money, for example, $300 to use as they please (for example, have a party or purchase a microwave oven). You may also invite departments to submit ideas for improvements that enhance the user friendliness of the department but cost money. The winning department gets the money needed to implement the change. These kinds of contests reinforce a customer-oriented mind set on the part of employees and also reward the team.

Once you have settled on the type of contest to hold, you have to go about selecting a prize for the winners. To amass tangible goodies to use as rewards, ask your local merchants to donate their products or services. Their contributions can benefit them as much as you, if you publicize their contributions. Figure 14-8 shows an example of a letter you could send to potential contributors.

Figure 14-7. Rules for a Hospital Scavenger Hunt

HOSPITALITY™

**Scavenger Hunt
for Employees - Physicians - Volunteers**

The second of the HOSPITALity House Rules, "Does Someone Look Confused?" emphasizes the difficulty many people have finding their way around Community Hospital. Sometimes it's even hard for employees to know where every department is located. This **modified scavenger hunt** will test your ability to "find" different areas throughout the Hospital. You may even learn the location of areas you didn't know existed.

There are 20 areas to identify from the maps: 25 questions total. Use this answer sheet and the maps attached to participate in the game. The 20 numbers on the maps represent department locations. Record the name of each of the departments next to the corresponding number below. It you are unsure of where a department is located, feel free to "scavenge" the area for a sign on the department door that will verify the accuracy of your answer.

It will be worth your while to be sure all your responses are correct because (1) you will be eligible for a grand prize drawing and (2) most important, you will be better able to give correct directions to persons who need assistance.

The winner, whose entry is drawn from all correct entries, will be "directed" to Mr. Corley's office to receive a gift certificate for one night's stay at the city's newest downtown hotel, Embassy Suites, that is good for up to four family members. This prize represents Community's commitment to the hospitality extended to all our guests, including patients, visitors, doctors, volunteers, and fellow employees. Good luck!

1) _____	11) _____
2) _____	12) _____
3) _____	13) _____
4) _____	14) _____
5) _____	15) _____
6) _____	16) _____
7) _____	17) _____
8) _____	18) _____
9) _____	19) _____
10) _____	20) _____

21) At what intersection is CHI-North located? _____
22) Where is the newest of the four Medchecks located? _____
23) The Arthritis Unit is located in Building _____, _____ Floor.
24) What department is located in the "little white house" on the SE corner of the hospital property? _____
25) The Hyperbaric Oxygen (HBO) Department is located in Building _____, _____ Floor.

Name: _____ Department: _____

Place your completed form in the blue box just inside the cafeteria door by Sunday, July 21, to participate. The maps are yours to keep for future use.

Figure 14-8.   Example of a Letter Asking for Donations of Prizes to Be Awarded to Contest Winners

---

Jane Doe, Manager
Public Relations
Anywhere Hotel
Address
City, State, Zip

Dear Ms. Doe:

We at Community General Memorial Hospital are engaged in a far-reaching effort to improve our services to patients.

As one part of our service excellence strategy, we are staging a contest on "Reducing Noise." All of our 3,000-plus employees are invited to submit entries on how to reduce both mechanical and human noise. To provide an incentive to entrants, we want to award prizes to the employees with the three best ideas.

Will you donate an escape weekend, a special meal for two, or some other goody we can offer as a prize in our contest? We will publicize your contribution widely in our hospital newsletter (circulation 6,000).

Since our contest begins in one month, I look forward to your response to our request. Thank you very much for your consideration.

Sincerely,

Giva Little
Director of Prize Solicitation

Events and Celebrations

Another way to remind, reinforce, and refresh is through special events and celebrations. For example, you may have an annual "Patient First Day" or a special speaker at a luncheon for middle managers. Here are descriptions of a few possibilities:

- *Be it resolved.* Pat Wright of Baptist Medical Center in Oklahoma City tells of the wonderful event her hospital conducted to renew employee commitment to their ongoing TLC Plus effort:
  —First, a written statement was developed on the hospital's purpose. The statement was called "Commitment to Caring."
  —Then, a press conference was arranged to cover the signing of the commitment by the hospital president and board.
  —At the ceremony, the signatures were affixed to a parchment scroll with the "Commitment to Caring" statement on top.
  —Afterward, at a reception, the employees signed the scroll and received a copy of the commitment and a special mug with a similar slogan.
  —The scroll was placed in a specially designed display case to be

installed in the hospital lobby. Copies were framed for hanging in every department and unit in the hospital.

—The "Commitment to Caring" statement was reproduced as a full-page ad for the local newspaper.

- *Entertainment through employee theater.* Several hospitals are rejuvenating customer relations thinking through original theater events developed by an employee theater troupe. At Einstein Medical Center, two theater extravaganzas, under Gail Scott's direction, boosted morale like nothing else Einstein ever tried.

In the original musical "Not Just Another Day," written by Gail Scott of the Einstein Consulting Group, hospital employees acted out three versions of one patient's hospital visit: first the horrible experience, then the ideal, and finally the achievable reality given the stresses on staff. "What's Good about Now," another musical written by Gail Scott and Chris McGovern, tells the story of a disillusioned hospital employee who seeks employment in a baby food company and, in the process, rediscovers what it was that first attracted her to health care; she returns to her job with a new mind set toward her work and renewed vigor.

An article in the HOSPITALity newsletter requested volunteers with any special talents or just an interest in theater. After the production of a program called "Not Just Another Day," the following appeared in the newsletter to explain why theater was chosen as a means to reinforce customer relations principles:

> Since we've been developing HOSPITALity at Einstein, many of you have urged us to find unconventional ways to look at the deeper issues behind HOSPITALity . . . ways to make HOSPITALity come alive and bring out the human emotions. Theater seemed promising. It's also an express route for reaching staff. (You know what it's like trying to get away for an in-service!) Theater's a fast medium, rich with messages.
>
> In our first production, we wanted to look at the issues involved in constructive staff relations and to strengthen the human element in our patient care. In an atmosphere of entertainment, theater can enter safely into these difficult issues and open channels of communication. People in the audience often identify with situations based on their own experiences and feelings, and this is what makes it meaningful.
>
> Someone new to Einstein who saw the production said, "It seemed so right. I thought theater had been around here for 100 years."

- *Walk a Day in My Shoes.* Elizabeth Farnell, R.N., director of nursing at Baptist Memorial Hospital in Memphis, Tennessee, developed this inspiring program that has doctors and nurses trading places for a day. They accompany one another on their rounds in order to better understand and appreciate each other's responsibilities. This program is now an annual event. Figure 14-9 shows the press release announcing the program.

□ Systemwide Refresher Programs

Although targeted-training experiences like those discussed in chapter 10 refresh customer relations skills, systemwide refresher programs that keep employees informed and address the organization's issues of the moment are extremely important. Many hospitals conduct one refresher program systemwide every six months. For instance, once a year, they conduct an update about the organization's progress, challenges, and success strategies and the part of employees in a winning formula. In this session, employee perceptions of customer relations strengths and weaknesses are solicited, and the objectives and plans for improvements communicated. Then, six months later, a second refresher is held on co-worker relationships, professional renewal, sales skills for employees, problem solving to improve patient satisfaction, complaint handling, or whatever other skills or organizationwide issues that a needs assessment has shown merit attention.

Film festivals can also be used to refresh systemwide efforts. People will come voluntarily if you promote the films actively, hold them at lunchtime so people can bring their lunch, or show them before or after work or in a cluster (one after another) at a social gathering where refreshments are served. Good possibilities for such a festival include:

- "Caring ... It Makes a Difference" and "Sometimes ... It's Harder to Care" from the American Hospital Association, 211 E. Chicago Ave., Chicago, IL 60611, 312/280-6030
- "A Gift from Mrs. Timm" and "Who Cares" from the Dartnell Corporation, 4660 Ravenswood Ave., Chicago, IL 60640, 312/561-4000
- "You Make the Difference" and "You Are This Hospital" from the Einstein Consulting Group, York and Tabor Roads, Philadelphia, PA 19141, 215/456-7065

Figure 14-9. Press Release Announcing the "Walk a Day in My Shoes" Program

Release:

Immediate

Contact:

Roy Jennings, director
Office of Communications
(901) 522-4324

MEMPHIS—Physicians and nurses at Baptist Memorial Hospital will be walking in each other's shoes during the next two weeks, a role exchange that promises to benefit the 60,000 patients who are treated at the facility each year.

From Sept. 19 through Sept. 30, "Walk a Day in My Shoes" will involve 54 physicians and 54 nurses observing each other during a normal workday.

"Our goal is to enhance the feeling of mutual respect and understanding that leads to better patient care," says Toni Pittman, R.N., coordinator of nurse recruitment for Baptist Memorial.

"Walk a Day in My Shoes" was coined by nursing director Elizabeth Farnell and stems from a successful program implemented more than a year ago in the 3,000-member nursing department at the hospital. That program involves nurses from various units swapping positions in order to experience firsthand and gain insight into the workings of other nursing areas.

"We are hearing that because Baptist is so big (1,500 beds at the medical center alone), nurses felt isolated on their individual units and not a part of the mainstream of nursing," Ms. Pittman says. "With the job swap program, they're better able to see the whole picture."

For instance, nurses from an intensive care unit and those from a general nursing floor switched positions and were able to follow how their care of a particular patient fit into his overall treatment from the time he was admitted critically ill to when he went home, Ms. Pittman says.

As well as improving patient care, the new program is expected to enhance physician-nurse communications, create an environment for collaboration, and create a positive climate for solving problems when they do occur, Ms. Pittman says.

Physicians from the active medical staff were asked to participate by the nursing staffs on the individual floors. A number of physicians were added to the program after hearing about it and asking to be included.

All three units of the hospital—the Medical Center, East, and Regional Rehabilitation Center—will participate.

(continued)

Figure 14-9. *(continued)*

> The day for a physician-nurse team will begin at 6:45 a.m. when nurses' morning report is held. The team will be involved in all phases of each member's day, from planning, preparing medications, informal and formal patient teaching, time spent making telephone calls, visiting patients (including in the physician's office), committee meetings, and the emergencies that occur daily for both.
>
> After the two weeks, participants will hold a dinner meeting to discuss and evaluate their day's "walk," Ms. Pittman says.

Reprinted with permission of Baptist Memorial Hospital, Memphis, Tennessee

☐ Tell the Public

You should brag about your strategy for service excellence and your customer relations orientation *after, and only after,* your strategy is in place and you have confidence in it. Issue a press release that calls public attention to your efforts. Invite media people in to see program components. Offer to appear on local talk shows. Call attention to your organization's emphasis on the quality of human interactions between patients and staff. Stress the service orientation of your hospital. The public likes to hear this.

☐ Final Suggestions

In your efforts to maintain, refresh, and advance awareness and skills related to service excellence, take the following precautions:

- *Don't fail the "taste test."* Make sure that any visual items you develop are tasteful within a health care environment. In their eagerness to develop eye-catching, attention-getting visuals and events, some hospitals have forgotten to examine their goods and ideas from the points of view of their customers. For example, one hospital kicked off its program with a big reception for all employees in the hospital's front lobby. They hired a person in a gorilla suit to entertain. In walked distraught family members on their way to visit their dying mother. Naturally, they were horrified at the insensitive carnival environment.
- *Don't fail the "credibility test."* Some posters, for instance, look great to the public, but employees know they aren't "true" and so feel disgusted with the people who created them. They blame the

new "P.R. mentality" and concern for "image" at any cost and call people's attention to what they perceive as hypocrisy on the part of the administration. Make sure the messages in your awareness campaigns, newsletters, and the like are truthful.

- *Avoid the machine-gun approach.* In their enthusiasm to produce refresher programs and visual campaigns, many customer relations coordinators and committees develop an ambitious, many-faceted campaign and institute it too rapidly. Then, their creative source and steam run dry. Space out your strategies for grabbing attention and refreshing commitment and motivation into a long-term, gradual, step-by-step, patient approach. Make the flavor last.
- *Don't delegate to the artists.* You probably have a public relations department or someone who designs your house publications, publicity, and campaigns. Be careful not to delegate customer relations campaigns to these talented people without the substantial involvement of the regular folks in your facility. The more broadly you involve employees at large and your task force members, the more ownership and stake people will have in every facet of your strategy, and the less likely you are to be accused of using a cosmetic approach.
- *Speaking of cosmetics.* If you don't have a solid strategy in place, don't do awareness campaigns and media events. Your employees and the public who accuse you of cosmetic image manipulation will be right. Build a strong foundation. Once it's built, brag, but be careful not to brag before you've built the base and seen results.

So many organizational priorities and everyday job demands compete for people's attention. To sustain a focus on service excellence so that a customer-oriented mind set guides employee behavior, you need to stubbornly resist letting your service excellence priority grow stale. An ongoing, varied, thoughtful agenda of reminders, refreshers, and attention grabbers keeps awareness high and deepens people's sensitivity to the breadth and depth of service excellence.

□Part Three

Operational Strategies

Planning for Service Excellence

"Young man, you certainly have a great gift. No matter
what they say about you, you have developed a unique skill.
Tell me," she said, "how did you get to be such a champion
shooter?"

The boy answered, "There's nothing to it. First you
shoot, and then you draw the target."

□   □   □

Having lost sight of our objective, we redoubled our efforts.
—Old Adage

□ Three-Stage Planning Process

If you ask around, you'll find many hospitals that launched customer
relations programs that yielded disappointing results. In some cases,
the necessary commitment was lacking. However, many hospitals
launched strategies before they were ready. They became impatient.
Excited and eager about the promise and possibilities, they initiated
customer relations with *inadequate planning*.

Planning for service excellence needs to be meticulous and

comprehensive and thoughtful. You need to make sure your foundation is strong before constructing the edifice itself. The goal of planning is to ensure that your strategy is carefully tailored to fit your organization's current realities and its problems, culture, and people.

If you have no strategy yet or if you feel you need to regroup or regenerate your strategy, institute a three-stage planning process:

- *Stage 1: Take the pulse of your organization.* What are its competitive position, image, culture, and norms? Also, what's the status of service excellence?
- *Stage 2: Characterize your employee population.* Identify the segments or subgroups of your employee population.
- *Stage 3: Identify components of a best-fit strategy that address the needs and concerns of every employee segment.* Motivate each segment and take steps to anticipate and minimize their resistance.

☐ Stage 1. Take the Pulse of Your Organization.

Investigate the competitive position, image, and organizational culture and norms of your institution that bear on your strategy for service excellence. Use various methods: first use your patient representatives, who are already close to your customers, and your patient questionnaire results, which undoubtedly contain a wealth of information. Then expand into an institutional audit that answers the following questions on competitive position, image, organizational culture and norms, administration, staff, and physicians:

- *On competitive position:*
  —Exactly how has your organization been doing financially? Are revenues up or down? Is volume up or down? Are donations up or down? What are the trends? To what are these trends attributed?
  —How serious are your financial problems? What is the profit-and-loss picture?
  —What are the population and economic trends affecting your organization? What trends are affecting reimbursement and demographics? What are the economic conditions in your local area?
  —What is your patient mix and the implications of reimbursement based on this mix?
  —What is the nature of the competition? Who are the old and new providers of similar services? What are your competitors' strategies? Who's winning and why?

—How worried or confident are administrators, trustees, and employees about your organization's financial health?

● *On image:*

—How does the public perceive your organization and its competitors? What kind of reputation does your organization really have?

—How does the community characterize your organization's strengths and weaknesses, especially in terms of the quality of service and customer relations provided?

—How do professionals perceive your institution?

—How do staff, patients, physicians, administrators, and trustees rate your services and people?

—What are the recurrent complaints?

—Specifically, how do various users of your services characterize the behavior of your work force?

● *On organizational culture and norms:*

—How would you describe the corporate culture of your facility? Is it friendly, supportive, open, caring, impersonal, cold, unfriendly, everyone for themselves, or other?

—What are the prevailing attitudes employees hold toward one another, toward top management, toward physicians, toward first-line supervisors, and toward their jobs?

—In the past, how have employees responded to efforts to involve them in making the organization more successful? To what extent does the organization have a ready constituency of employees interested in helping the organization achieve an improved competitive position?

—How have new programs been initiated? To what extent were employees involved? How are new programs received?

—In terms of customer relations, what standards do employees maintain by their behavior? What standards does peer pressure support? To what extent are people consumer oriented? What cultural idiom is projected by prevailing cultural or ethnic norms?

—What resistance to change do different people perceive?

—What feelings do customers experience when they walk into your facility? Why?

—How much do people trust one another? Why?

—How do employees feel about working here? Is there a lot of turnover? Why or why not? Is productivity high or low?

● *On the administration:*

—To what extent does your CEO manage by "walking around"? How visible is your administrative team?

—Does everyone in your organization know who the CEO is and

also who the top executives are by name?

—How regularly does the administration communicate with all staff either through letters, newsletters, announcements, regular meetings, and so forth?

—How regularly does the administration meet with department heads to update them on marketing direction, competition, new programs, fiscal health, and problems that need solutions?

—How frequent and successful are morale-boosting events, like talent shows, cafeteria bashes, birthdays off, team competition, and friendly interdepartmental events?

—How stable is top management, or do the key leaders change frequently?

● *On the staff:*

—To what extent do people smile and talk to one another in the halls and elevators, or do they move about with impassive faces?

—How much pride do people take in their work space?

—How proud are people of the medical tradition in which they participate? Do they show their pride by working in clean, crisp clothing and acting in a professional manner?

—To what extent are staff encouraged to participate in decision making to make their work environment better? Are suggestions and innovations encouraged?

—Does the hospital have a newsletter that highlights staff achievements and news?

—Do people sit together in the cafeteria and talk to one another?

—How well do departments cooperate for the good of the whole?

—How much do people take initiative, or is the attitude that "it's not my job" rampant?

● *On physicians:*

—How much cooperation exists between staff physicians and referring physicians?

—How much cooperation exists between physicians, nurses, and other staff?

—To what extent are referring physicians extended the courtesies common to guests, such as convenient admitting, access to patient information, accessible parking, and comfortable, well-equipped lounges?

To get information that is truly useful in planning, use a variety of methods to get diverse points of view. Some methods worth considering are:

● Focus groups with diverse employees

- Interviews with top and middle managers
- Extensive, ongoing surveys of patients
- Interviews with patients, physicians, visitors, and employee "opinion leaders"
- First-hand observation

☐ Stage 2. Characterize Your Employees

To develop a strategy that works for everyone, a working definition of *everyone* has to be achieved. Specifically, employee segments need to be identified according to their attitudinal predispositions so that you can tailor your motivational strategies to them.

You can accomplish this segmentation through observations, interviews, focus groups, and surveys. The objective at this stage is to understand the extent of the skill or behavior problems you have and to realize the attitudes through which employees can be expected to screen any new strategy or program aimed at behavior or attitude change. If you ignore these attitudes, or fail to consider them explicitly in your plan, you won't be prepared to prevent or handle constructively any resistance that's likely to emerge.

In this stage, ask the following questions:

- How do employees behave toward your customers? Is rudeness, for instance, mainly found in certain departments or among people in particular jobs? What behavior standards are set by the personal behavior of administrators and middle managers?
- How do different employee segments characterize your institution's service problems? For instance, do nurses think that some nurses do not extend themselves to customers because they are not being paid enough? Do housekeepers think that some housekeepers are not as hospitable as they could be because they have not been made aware of what is really expected of them in interactions with customers?
- What attitudinal predispositions characterize different segments of the work force when they are confronted with the idea of a change and with the idea of customer relations?
- What obstacles to change do different groups perceive?

☐ Stage 3. Identify Strategic Components

After you've taken stock of your organization's competitive position and organizational environment for change and examined the attitudes, values, and behavior of your multifaceted target population, you can design your strategy based on sound information. You may design your strategy yourself or locate outside resources that can help you develop a *best-fit, institutionwide strategy* that incorporates all that you have learned about your organization's reality and the people involved. A best-fit strategy is needed because your strategy has to affect heterogeneous employee groups all at once. Unfortunately, you can't hold Monday workshops for cynics, Tuesday workshops for enthusiasts, and Wednesday workshops for the people insulted by what they expect to be a "charm-school" approach to customer relations. Your people have diverse feelings and perspectives, and your strategy needs to speak to these effectively. The whole situation is not easy because what works to motivate some people runs the risk of alienating others.

To design a best-fit strategy tailored to your diverse employee population, consider these steps:

- Characterize segments of your employee population according to their attitudinal predispositions toward a customer relations strategy.
- Clarify each employee segment's definition of the customer relations problem in your organization.
- Generate carefully the messages suited to motivate each segment to improve their behavior, given their attitude toward and definition of your organization's problems.
- Design special strategy components to communicate the message that is appropriate to each employee segment.
- Refine each strategy component so that it does not simultaneously alienate or trigger resistance among other segments.

Let's illustrate this process with an example from the early days of customer relations planning at Albert Einstein Medical Center. Figure 15-1 summarizes the results of the planning process (Martin Goldsmith and Wendy Leebov, *Healthcare Management Review*, 1986 Spring, 11[2]:87-88). This tedious, complex, and thorough planning process was the force that jet-propelled Einstein's strategy to early success.

Once you've done all the groundwork, consider each pillar of service excellence discussed in part II and generate strategies for strengthening each pillar. Be sure that the strategies you devise consider the feelings and behavior of your target groups. You'll find more about planning for follow-through in chapter 19.

Figure 15-1. Structure for Designing a Best-Fit Strategy: An Example

Employee segment according to attitudes toward improving behavior toward hospital guests	How each employee segment defines the problem	Major message appropriate to this segment	Program component designed to convey this message
a. *Willing and able* (team players): "I will change, now that I know how important my behavior is." OR "I guess I could *do better. I'll try.*"	*"Other* people are uncooperative."	"We have a perplexing economic situation. You can help."	• Briefing on the economic situation. • Communication of explicit HOSPITALity expectations or House Rules.
b. *Willing and unable:* "I would change if I knew how."	"People don't know how to do what's expected."	"Here's how."	• Specialized training for people in position involving substantial public contact.
c. *Cooperative but distracted:* "I mean well; I would extend myself to guests more if I would think of it more often."	"I'm overworked; I have too much on my mind—too many pressures."	"We'll help you remember."	• Reminders in the environment (newsletters, posters, special events, training for supervisors on giving ongoing recognition and feedback).
d. *Resigned:* "I will if I must."	"It's not me. It's the doctors. But go ahead. Lay something else on us."	"We now have explicit standards. All are expected to meet them. Those who don't will suffer consequences. This applies to all—you, your coworkers, your supervisors, and doctors."	• Communication of explicit standards. • Program for supervisors on how to hold people to new higher standards using motivation techniques and the discipline process. • Programs that communicate explicit expectations to physicians.

(continued)

251

Figure 15-1. *(continued)*

Employee segment according to attitudes toward improving behavior toward hospital guests	How each employee segment defines the problem	Major message appropriate to this segment	Program component designed to convey this message
e. *Oppressed:* "Everyone needs to get their act together. Then, I'll think about it."	"Other people mistreat us. If they would treat us right, we'd treat them and patients right."	"New standards apply to all (administrators, you, your supervisors, and doctors). If everyone waits for everyone else to change, we have a stalemate. Of course, you are not the *cause* of our hospital's problems, but we need you to be a part of the solution."	• Opportunity to vent feelings and problems. • Suggestion boxes and other outlets and suggestions. • A broader perspective on the hospital's economic problems and resulting pressures on everyone involved.
f. *Resentful:* "This is cosmetic! What about the deeper problems? Why do they go unsolved year after year? I'll cooperate if you make my life less miserable."	"Working conditions are unfair. There have been problems here for years. Why didn't they solve these problems? Now they're pointing the finger at us! The bosses don't care about us employees or our input."	"Certainly, we need to change other things here beyond employee behavior, and we are. Here's how—and to make headway on these and other problems we're establishing more accessible routes through which you can bring problems to light and suggest solutions."	• Opportunity to vent feelings and problems. • Suggestion boxes. • Employee rap sessions. • Methods for feeding back to employees actions taken as a result of their suggestions.
g. *Cynics:* "Why bother? This is just another program. It's hopeless."	"It's the times we're living in and the kinds of people we have here."	Communicate the power of the self-fulfilling prophecy. "If you expect an effort to fail, you'll probably be proven right. If we decide to believe change is possible, we can make it happen."	• Honesty about hospital economics. • Motivational appeal on the power of the self-fulfilling prophecy. • Sharing of data on how positively hospital guests already perceive employees.

(continued)

Figure 15-1. *(continued)*

Employee segment according to attitudes toward improving behavior toward hospital guests	How each employee segment defines the problem	Major message appropriate to this segment	Program component designed to convey this message
h. *Rebellious/Refusing:* "I won't change, and you can't make me."	"The administration always blames everything on us. I won't shape up. Let them shape up."	"If you don't meet expectations, you won't last here."	• Issue policy requiring conformity to explicit standards. • Train supervisors to deal with marginal employees and to use hospital's progressive discipline process.
i. *Insulted:* "I'm a professional! You want to *train* me to smile? How degrading!"	"The doctors and administrators are the problem . . . and the incredible pressure's on us."	"Of course, you already know how to be nice. You're a dedicated professional. We're asking you to *consistently* do what you know is best. This will gain you the respect you deserve. If you can achieve *distinction* or excellence in our treatment of hospital guests, our hospital (and you) will be respected more and our competitive position improved. This is how you help us succeed."	• Economic briefing, emphasizing the need to become superior, not just good, in our competitive environment. • Positive approach to motivating people; building on strengths; exploring the subtleties of behavior.

Reprinted from "Strengthening the Hospital's Market Position through Training," by Martin Goldsmith and Wendy Leebov, in *HealthCare Management Review*, 1986 Spring, 11(2):87-88. Reprinted with permission of Aspen Publishers, Inc. Copyright 1986.

☐ Final Suggestions

As you plan your strategy for service excellence, you should keep the following in mind:

- *Watch out for flashes in the pan.* You need to develop a long-range plan for service excellence that reassures your employees that the emphasis on service excellence is not a short-lived enthusiasm. This reassurance is especially important if your organization has a history of starting programs with a bang but then letting them fizzle. Show people a staged, carefully sequenced strategy that goes on year after year.
- *Start by clarifying your vision.* Remember this from *Alice in Wonderland*: " 'Cheshire Puss,' she [Alice] began, 'would you please tell me which way I ought to go from here?' 'That depends on where you want to get to,' said the cat." Be sure you know exactly where you want to go.
- *Involve a wide array of key people from the start.* Dwight Eisenhower said that plans are nothing, but planning is everything. Eisenhower knew what he was talking about when he emphasized the power that the planning process has in building commitment and in ensuring clarity of purpose and a shared sense of direction among people whose cooperation is key to making things happen.

The planning process is tedious and complex but also necessary. A good planning process is necessary if you want to develop a plan that minimizes resistance and maximizes results. As usual, prevention is easier than the cure and less costly. Consider the tedious, complex planning job as an investment that reduces false starts, dead ends, and risks and increases the chance that your vision will become reality.

□ **Chapter 16**

Staffing for Service Excellence

Even though customer relations is everybody's job, you still need to assign staff to hold your strategy together and propel it forward. If you're engaging in a full-fledged customer relations strategy, you need to make sure you have a large enough staff to carry out the complex functions that a full-scale strategy entails. No customer relations strategy can thrive unless it has at least one nameable human being whose job is to coordinate the strategy, another person providing support, and an active steering committee and subcommittees.

Who exactly do you need to carry out a comprehensive customer relations strategy?

- You need a *director, coordinator, or boss* who reports to a respected administrator with clout. This director, coordinator, or boss needs secretarial support. In reality, most "mortals" cannot serve this function *on top of* another full-time job unless their priorities are radically shifted or support staff added to help. In some situations, a dynamic team who devote part-time to the effort can manage a comprehensive strategy for service excellence.
- You need a strong, active customer relations *steering committee or task force.*
- You need *everyone*—administrators, managers, supervisors, and all other employees—to understand that customer relations is still *everyone's responsibility,* despite the fact that certain people have

been given overt responsibilities for coordinating customer relations activities.

Consider a coordinator, director, or boss. This person (or two persons) must be a leader in the hospital. He or she should report to an effective administrator with clout, a credible, respected administrator who can and will make things happen organizationally for the sake of service excellence. Unfortunately, some hospitals have given an ineffective administrator customer relations oversight because customer relations is a "soft" area. This kind of "oversight" can indeed prove to be an oversight of monumental proportions for the strategy. All too soon, the customer relations strategy can become just another weak program with a short life. Then, no wonder other administrators and many employees call the strategies a failure and disband them completely because they conclude, "You can't make headway with customer relations." In the quiet of the night, these people must know that the strategy never had a chance because the organization failed to put the necessary vision, push, and clout behind it.

Two nonfiction stories hopefully illuminate this point:

- *Story one:* In a medium-size hospital in the Southeast, a dynamite patient representative spearheads customer relations activities in her organization. She developed the committee, built grass-roots support, researched the state of the art, learned from other organizations' successes and failures, educated herself, and developed a plan after soliciting involvement and commitment from many people in the organization.

  The administration got excited about it and decided to commit resources. The vice-president for human resources saw the excitement among his colleagues. He saw that resources were being committed. He had an insight. He could expand his department's turf and work on a "hot-button" program if he could grab customer relations for his department. The result would be more status for his department in the organization.

  He found five other hospitals with the customer relations function in the human resources department and pressed his case. His colleagues were delighted. Seeing this vice-president enthusiastic for the first time in years, they agreed to give him responsibility for customer relations, hoping that he would at last do something with vigor.

  Remember the patient representative who did all the work, the one who had the vision, the one who amassed support. The vice-president didn't even invite her to serve on the committee. Do you suppose he was too threatened by her effectiveness and coworker support?

Can you guess the end of this tale? Customer relations started off with a whimper. The vice-president did not, you may be shocked to know, make good decisions about the content, scope, or extent of the strategy needed. After all, he had never really understood what makes a customer relations strategy successful, nor did he really care. The patient representative is still there, but she is angry that she was passed over, bitter that customer relations turned into a political tool, and disappointed that what could have been a meaningful program for both patients and staff never will be.

- *Story two:* In a large teaching hospital in the West, administrators decided to institute a serious long-term customer relations strategy. The person who researched the possibilities was their director of training. This director was competent and hard-working but not really liked by peers or administrators. Because the director was already going full-tilt on customer relations, the administrators followed the path of least resistance and let her oversee the customer relations strategy.

  She started up full-steam, but people didn't want to work with her because people didn't like her. She convened a committee, but the meetings were frustrating to people because she ran them in a rigid, plodding way.

  The customer relations strategy crawled forward, but the administrators and department heads and supervisors minimized their role because they habitually avoided working with the director. Finally, they concluded that the customer relations strategy was a disappointment, that it just didn't do what they hoped it would do for the organization. And they were right. The strategy was extremely weak because the administration was not making the courageous move it needed to make to get the strategy on a strong footing. They would have to work with or replace the director, hash out meaningful follow-up, and devote some of their own energies to the strategy. However, all they'll do is wish the director wasn't there, and the strategy will fade into oblivion.

These two stories illustrate staffing problems that played havoc with customer relations progress. Your organization's leadership must make sure that the staff for customer relations is not only *knowledgeable, respected, and experienced* in program management, but is also *good* at these jobs.

☐ Customer Relations in the Organizational Hierarchy

No particular place is the best place for customer relations across all organizations. The right home for it depends entirely on your organization's structure and politics. Some organizations locate the customer relations function within an existing department.

Others create a department of customer relations and then must decide to whom it should report. Some people say that customer relations should report directly to the CEO or at least to a key administrator.

The customer relations function can work successfully in the patient relations area or in departments of marketing, volunteer services, public relations, risk management, quality assurance, nursing, radiology, training, personnel, management engineering, and more. The key is not the department name. The key is that wherever you locate the coordination function for customer relations, you must put it in a supportive context so that it has primary, not secondary, importance. Also, it needs to be tied closely to a key administrator.

The best departmental home for customer relations should be:

- Clearly patient oriented
- Clearly able to devote resources to customer relations without creating a conflict of interest
- Filled with people who are credible from a customer relations point of view. For example, if the personnel department is notoriously out of touch with employee concerns, don't put the customer relations function there.
- Be willing to coordinate the strategy, but not carry it only on its own shoulders and thus destroy the potential of widespread employee involvement and infusion into the entire hospital culture.

Ideally, you would have a department of guest or customer relations that is staffed by people experienced in patient and physician advocacy as well as in troubleshooting for service excellence. The staff also includes people who are skilled in physician relations as well as people who do the administrative work. For many hospitals, this ideal will always be wishful thinking. The best they can do is to choose the "right" person as the coordinator of the customer relations activities and the strategy for service excellence.

□ The Right Coordinator

The coordinator is the orchestra conductor who coordinates the various players to sustain your strategy for service excellence. Continuing with the pillar metaphor, the coordinator is your contractor who coordinates people, committees, and subcommittees to ensure that together they build strong pillars to support customer relations.

What does a coordinator do? Figure 16-1 shows elements of an ideal job description for a customer relations coordinator. Some of these elements may already be part of existing positions. Few individuals could adequately fulfill all of these job responsibilities by themselves. Nevertheless, all the functions listed have to be served in some way, by either internal or external human resources.

Instead of creating a new position and posting or searching for the right person in the usual fashion, Charles O'Brien, administrator of Georgetown University Hospital in Washington, DC, tried an innovative approach to filling the job. Believing that a respected and senior Georgetown employee could best fill the coordinator's job, he advertised a one-year sabbatical. The winner would take a leave from his or her current position and serve as customer relations coordinator. The following are the criteria for the selection of the coordinator:

• The candidate should be able to articulate his or her understanding of the customer relations program, the importance of it, and his or her plans for implementing it throughout the hospital.
• The candidate must receive the endorsement of his or her supervisor, who must indicate how the candidate's present responsibilities would be handled if he or she were selected.
• The candidate must be able to demonstrate a proved ability in verbal and written communication skills.
• The candidate must be able to demonstrate good judgment, maturity, and an understanding of the operating systems of the hospital.
• The successful candidate must have significant managerial responsibility, including, but not limited to, that of a department head.

After a successful year on the job, the person selected by Charles O'Brien decided to stay on as the customer relations coordinator.

The customer relations coordinator is inevitably a booster and flak-catcher. A hospital always has some people who resist any new idea;

Figure 16-1. Job Description for the Customer Relations Coordinator

Major Job Responsibilities

1. Develops, coordinates, and evaluates the implementation of a long-range plan for improving patient, visitor, employee, and physician customer relations, including complex scheduling, writing correspondence and reports, recruiting of employees to act as workshop leaders, and related duties.

2. Creates and coordinates a long-term steering committee and several subcommittees to develop, implement, monitor, and troubleshoot key components of the customer relations strategy.

3. Develops and implements methods for monitoring staff concerns, obtaining staff input on problems, and feeding back responses and actions taken.

4. Develops and implements or works with other patient relations people to implement methods of:
   a. Monitoring patient, visitor, and physician satisfaction with various hospital practices and services.
   b. Serving as a catalyst in follow-up.
   c. Communicating results to appropriate parties.

5. Intervenes (along with other advocacy staff) to engage administrators and other key individuals and departments to solve problems that interfere with customer satisfaction.

6. Develops strategies that build employee morale and commitment to service excellence.

7. Conducts stand-up training sessions and speeches for employee groups, physicians, and physician office staff to build their customer relations skills. (This responsibility is not part of the job in every situation.)

8. Manages the time line for the customer relations strategy, by coordinating the work of various people and departments, including public relations, patient relations, physician relations, personnel, marketing, training and education, nursing, and others.

9. Handles other duties as required.

Requirements

1. College degree, with master's degree in human service area or service-related field preferred.

2. Excellent communication skills, including writing, speaking, counseling, and intergroup problem solving.

3. At least three years' experience in management, supervision, team building, training, and problem solving in a complex service organization.

4. Experience in health care setting in relevant job or experience in service industry.

5. Excellent organizational and project-management skills.

6. The energy, stamina, and persistence to be a change agent, and the ability to work independently.

some cooperative people who fail to keep their promise; some people who are raring to go and want more to do; and some people who see your director as a goody-two-shoes, Pollyanna, complaint department, cynic's respite, and lightning rod for every spark that flies between people. So in addition to the characteristics of an effective coordinator described so far, your coordinator also needs to have:

- Guts
- Thick skin
- Aplomb
- Acceptance
- Assertiveness
- Guts
- Flexibility
- Self-confidence
- Dogged, unflinching persistence
- Guts

At times, the coordinator is a shorthanded one-person band. When people are recruited, hired, or pinpointed for the coordinator's role, the need for almost heroic attention to detail is too often underplayed.

If you have a strategy in place, someone in your organization already has faced this reality firsthand. If not, here's a description of just a smattering of the details that most coordinators have to handle early on in their tenure. This example focuses *only* on *one* of many components in their overall work: preparation for the training of workshop facilitators. To prepare for training your workshop leaders, the coordinator has to:

- Organize and implement the process for selecting workshop leaders.
- Communicate the results of the leader-selection process to the leaders chosen and not chosen and to the rest of the staff.
- Schedule the training for your workshop leaders and notify the leaders and their supervisors of the time involved.
- Reserve adequate, consistent, reliable, conducive space.
- Order lunch and morning and afternoon refreshments.
- Arrange for audiovisual equipment; make sure it works and is there on time.
- Prepare and duplicate materials.
- Develop a typed list of workshop leaders' names, departments, and telephone numbers.
- Arrange for an administrator to visit the training session and address the group.

- Ease prospective leaders' concerns and fears and last-minute cold feet.
- Participate in the training sessions fully, working to develop a supportive relationship with the workshop leaders.
- Arrange a special time for workshop leaders to learn how to use the audiovisual equipment; allow time for practice.
- Become expert in the audiovisual equipment so you can troubleshoot when needed.
- Come to training sessions with the workshop schedule and a method of matching workshop leaders to sessions.
- Plan for the recognition of workshop leaders.
- Develop frequent, nurturing support systems for workshop leaders.

These details or subtasks are just a few of the details or subtasks associated with only one small facet of the coordinator's role, that of preparing workshop leaders for employee workshops. The list of details and subtasks associated with the workshops themselves is much longer, and the same is true for every component of the customer relations strategy.

The customer relations coordinator has to be a special, committed, multitalented person or team. You need to do all you can to make sure people appreciate the complexity of the role and the extreme dedication, stamina, and skill that the person or persons who fill that job must well have.

☐ Steering Committee

A customer relations steering committee is essential. You may already have such a customer relations advisory committee, steering committee, or task force. If so, you may want to make sure you have the right people on it. If you have no such committee, consider developing one. Without such a committee, your coordinator will surely feel isolated, swamped, and perhaps powerless.

What can a committee do? It can do plenty if it's set up well, consists of the right people, and has leadership pushing, pulling, and supporting its efforts. A committee can:

- Guide, monitor, and support your customer relations strategy.
- Take operational responsibility for key facets of your overall strategy so your director does not drown in all the work.
- Build a broad base of support among influential people who can advocate for decisions and resources needed to make your strategy successful.

The Committee's Main Tasks

The functions reflected in the 10 pillars of customer relations excellence mentioned in chapter 4 and described in detail in part II need to be accomplished with the leadership of your steering committee members. Many hospitals develop 10 subcommittees that closely parallel the 10 pillars of customer relations excellence. Each subcommittee is chaired by a member of the steering committee and consists of people with knowledge, experience, and credibility related to that subcommittee's function.

Among the specific tasks that need to be done are these:

- *Input and evaluation.* A subcommittee needs to develop and implement a plan for pretesting and posttesting the perceptions that employees, physicians, patients, and visitors have of customer relations. Also, ongoing sources of information from your customers need to be developed to guide your organization's strategy.
- *Revision of personnel policies and accountability systems.* A subcommittee that includes a key person in the personnel department needs to build customer relations standards and expectations into personnel policies that include basic policy, job descriptions, and performance appraisal. Also, standards for screening and hiring staff for their potential in customer relations need to be formulated, approved, and instituted.
- *Physician involvement.* A subcommittee needs to take responsibility for developing a plan for involving physicians in customer relations. This responsibility involves the design, scheduling, and promotion of an appropriate intervention, given your facility's medical staff structure and politics.
- *Communication devices to keep service excellence themes alive.* A subcommittee needs to develop and implement a strategic plan for the written promotion of service excellence in your existing house publications and in any new publications developed for this purpose, and on T-shirts, on posters, and so forth.
- *Problem solving and complaint clearinghouse.* A subcommittee needs to make sure that the hospital has adequate systems for soliciting, reviewing, and acting on complaints and suggestions from every customer group. Hopefully, you already have patient representatives or others collecting data, analyzing it, and funneling it to those people who can act on it. If you already have such individuals, then the committee's responsibility involves being sure that systems for information gathering are adequate, that information is fed into a problem-solving and action structure, that complaints are tracked well and resulting actions noted, and that the people concerned are informed.

- *New employee orientation.* A person or subcommittee needs to develop a strong customer relations component to be included in new-employee orientation. This component needs to orient new people to the strong priority the hospital places on customer relations, to communicate clear and explicit expectations for employee behavior, and to motivate new people to do all they can for the hospital.
- *Staff development, training, and job-specific skill building.* A subcommittee needs to identify job-specific personnel groups that need skill building in order to be excellent in customer relations. They then need to develop a long-range plan to use inside or outside resources to involve these groups in skill development.
- *Recognition and reward.* A subcommittee needs to survey existing recognition and reward strategies and then, based on their findings, strengthen or design new options and programs.
- *Employee as customer.* This subcommittee needs to focus on addressing employee needs for belonging, job enrichment, accomplishment, participation, and fun. Some hospitals focus this responsibility more specifically on developing morale-boosting events, and one even calls its subcommittee the "Fun Committee."
- *Refreshers, reminders, and attention grabbers.* A subcommittee needs to begin working on follow-through ideas, refresher programs, special events, and other methods for maintaining employee awareness and commitment.

Composition of Your Steering Committee

The question of who should be on your steering committee is controversial. Paul Murphy of the Einstein Consulting Group claims that the best committees have as half of their members key managers with critical components of the customer relations strategy in their areas of expertise (for example, a training specialist who can help with training programs and a personnel expert who can help improve accountability devices). The other half, Paul says, should be the *lunatic fringe,* the visionaries and mavericks at all levels of the organization who are willing to stick their necks out to achieve service excellence. He even thinks that the biggest maverick should lead the committee, because of that person's energy, drive, and unwillingness to let the strategy fall dormant.

This view has merit. Whether you agree or not, certain facts are clear about the composition of an effective committee. Your steering committee needs to include:

- *People from various departments.* Having people in departments

most tied to each of the 10 pillars is helpful but not essential, because these content experts can be on the subcommittee designed to make specific changes related to their areas.
- *People from various status levels.* Some people say to include only managers. Others say to include at least two people who are front-line employees to keep the committee respectful and honest.
- *At least one, or more, influential administrator.*
- *Passionately committed people.*

Also, the committee should be voluntary. Nothing is more paralyzing than having a customer relations steering committee filled with people who serve begrudgingly, who do all they can to be unable to attend meetings, and who have no steam for following through on their task commitments. Voluntary service is essential. Have the committee set attendance and activity-level standards so that people must quit unless they hold up their ends.

Typical committees include a subset of people in the following positions, if these poeple qualify as mavericks who bring sufficient energy and vision to the job:

- Customer relations coordinator
- Director of personnel or human resources
- Influential, interested member of administrative team
- Respected nursing management person
- Patient representative
- Person involved in employee training and education
- Key person from public relations area
- Key person from marketing area
- Influential physician or person in physician-liaison position or both
- Four or five other influential employees from service areas (for example, dietary, nursing, and environmental service) and "backroom" areas (for example, labs or storeroom)

The chairperson of the steering committee may be appointed by the administration or selected by the committee itself.

In short, enthusiasts must be mixed with people who have the authority to make things happen, in case these categories are nonoverlapping. If you don't have power in the group, the enthusiasts fast become frustrated cynics.

Committee Start-Up

After you decide who should be on your steering committee and who should be the chairperson, move immediately into action. If you don't, you set the stage for slow movement, not to mention procrastination and avoidance. The following should be done at your first meeting:

- Invite people to share their personal visions of service excellence.
- Clearly delineate the mission of each subcommittee.
- Choose the chairpersons of each subcommittee.
- Set dates for the next four to six meetings and have people mark the dates in their calendars.
- Give clear homework to be done before the next meeting. Specifically, ask every subcommittee chairperson to answer these questions by the second meeting:
  —Who do you think should be on your subcommittee?
  —What are the specific objectives of your subcommittee?
  —What's already happening in the organization that could help you accomplish your subcommittee's task?
  —What's a draft version of a time line and action plan for meeting your objectives? Develop a rough mockup for the larger committee to review for the purposes of getting on the same wavelength.
  Chairpeople don't have to answer these questions completely, but looking for answers pushes them forward and also tests their willingness to serve as active, productive subcommittee chairpeople. If a committee member is going to be inactive early on, you had best find out so that you can replace that person and not let him or her drag your committee down.

At your second meeting, have each person present their plan to the group and share reactions. The purpose is to clarify the mandate and strategy for each subcommittee. At future meetings, people report on their progress and help one another solve problems related to carrying out their jobs well and on time. Also, the entire committee reviews results to date and begins the troubleshooting and follow-through process. At least once every six months, the committee should go through a team-building experience to help people maintain their cohesion and energy for the job.

Paul Murphy identifies additional opportunities, or critical points, for productive and purposeful committee involvement. He claims that the coordinator can keep the committee motivated and useful by involving them actively at these key points:

- *Early on.* The committee should be convened to develop its own vision, mission statement, and sense of direction. They should review the 10 pillars and generate a plan to build each one strongly.

The group should present its vision and its plan to the administrative team and should state the resources committee members think are needed to make their vision and plan happen.

- *Focus group.* The committee should be its own focus group or think tank in its analysis of the organization's service strengths and weaknesses. It should begin to target specific areas and problems that need special attention.
- *Personal contributions.* The committee should build cohesion and a sense of team. Individuals should be asked to identify contributions they can and want to make. They should also state what they need from the group and from others in order to carry out their responsibilities fully and with support.
- *Pilot the workshops.* Ideally committee members should be participants in pilot tests of employee workshops at an early-enough stage so that they can give feedback on the style, message, and content of the program.
- *Training of workshop leaders.* If you are training employees to conduct workshops, the committee should make a short presentation to the workshop leaders to share with them the committee's mission, hopes, expectations, and support.
- *Postworkshop meetings with workshop leaders.* After the workshops are complete, the committee should convene the workshop leaders and pump them for all they learned about organizational needs and problems and for their recommendations for priority follow-through goals.
- *Regrouping after workshops.* Having heard the workshop leaders' perspectives, the committee needs to once again plan its strategy and to identify what exactly needs to be done to move the organization forward toward customer relations excellence. Also, after the workshops, many committees ask some of the workshop leaders to become members of subcommittees.

☐ Employees as Workshop Leaders

If, as part of your plan, employees are trained to conduct workshops for your employee population, here are a few hints about the characteristics of those employees who have proved to be the best workshop leaders for customer relations:

- *Status mix.* Select people from all walks of hospital life, union and nonunion, various levels and departments and positions, clinical and nonclinical.
- *Diversity mix.* Select diverse people by race, ethnic group, gender,

and age so that the diversity of your work force is reflected in the selections.

- *Opinion leaders.* Select people who have the respect and ear of their peers because when these people talk, others listen. Look for the *informal leaders* of your organization.
- *Communicators.* Select people who are willing (even though they may be nervous) to talk, write, and read in front of large groups.
- *Enthusiasm and charisma.* Select people who are outspoken and enthusiastic.
- *Role models.* Select people who exemplify the spirit and skills of excellent customer relations toward patients, doctors, visitors, and coworkers.
- *Gregarious, outgoing people.*
- *Open-minded, nondefensive people.* Select open-minded, non-defensive people because they will need to handle resistance and hostility.
- *Realists.* Select people who are aware of, but not debilitated by, the organization's problems. Select optimists, but not Pollyannas.

Caution and care in selecting workshop leaders pay off in your employees' acceptance of the customer relations message.

☐ Advice to All Key Players

However you staff for customer relations excellence, you need involvement from a wide range of people who become stakeholders, and these people have to be the right people. In her presentation to the American Society of Healthcare Education and Training in June 1985, Katie Buckley of the Einstein Consulting Group specified *nine musts* for all the people who staff your customer relations function in any way, from full-time staff to committee and subcommittee members.

- *Act the expert and educate others.* Given the time, investment, and responsibility, your key players are the experts in customer relations relative to others in your organization. Who else but these staff can then educate administrators about what it takes to get results. Too often administrators know what they want, but they don't know what it takes to get it. Administrators need to understand the scope and depth of your strategy, but they won't without a catalytic process by concerned people.
- *Establish a vision and let it lead you and hang on to it through thick and thin.* Customer relations has to be a long-term concern. Therefore, it requires faith, endurance, commitment, and vision.

To sustain momentum, the vision needs to be shared by a nucleus of visionary people who drive others and who overcome the inevitable setbacks and hurdles. As layoffs and cutbacks, traumatic change, leadership, and other problems take their toll on your organization and people, your customer relations visionaries need to help people see the light at the end of the tunnel.

- *Use your integrity instinct.* Your key people need to tune into their instincts to test whether your strategy for service excellence has integrity and is ethically justifiable, honest, and credible. This instinct is what tells people that you must somehow involve physicians. This instinct is what tells you to take seriously and act on employee perceptions of problems and obstacles to customer relations. Your integrity instinct propels your key players to spell out to administration what they need to do to make your effort credible and effective.

- *Know the patient.* Customer relations strategies are hollow unless driven by a few people's firsthand knowledge and experience with patients. You can't do all your planning sitting around a table. At every major turn, your key players must tune in on the patient to see if you're on the right path. Hear their complaints, criticisms, and frustrations. Understand their anxieties and fears. Witness their smiles and tears. Without personalizing customer relations through empathy, customer relations remains an empty concept lacking in emotion, persuasion, and drive.

- *Advocate for the patient.* Key players have several roles: educator, mediator with administration, change agent, cheerleader, taskmaster, and the like. The core role, however, needs to be that of *advocate* for better patient care. The advocate role is your foundation when negotiating with administration for resources and support.

- *Know the employee.* In addition to empathizing with patients, your key players also have to empathize with fellow employees. They need to break through the attitude-problem syndrome and see employee frustrations and concerns as legitimate. To do so, they have to get firsthand information about coworkers' feelings toward customer relations, their perceptions of your organization's problems, and the dynamics and pressures that make their work life difficult. Key players need to imagine themselves working eight hours a day, five days a week in a dead-end job, being treated as a third-class citizen in a hierarchical structure that mitigates against common courtesy and human decency, running themselves ragged answering phones, righting wrongs, working double shifts, handling mounds of paperwork, and doing all this for a supervisor who isn't friendly or respectful. The ability of your key players to "step into the shoes" of every employee helps them avoid conveying through strategy components punitive messages. Instead, they can build the more appropriate and motivating theme of empowerment into your customer relations approach.

- *Work with resistance positively.* An avalanche of resistance is usually inevitable when customer relations programs are begun. If your key players treat resistance as inevitable and informative, they can make it a catalyst to developing a more credible and widely accepted customer relations approach.
- *Expand your image of what you can do for your organization.* Customer relations strategies reach deep within the organization's systems. To realize the potential, leaders of your effort need an expanded image of who they are and what they can contribute. This image allows them to break loose from customary and traditional roles.
- *Have the courage to care.* Customer relations pioneering takes endurance. The monster machine of technology and bureaucracy can seem insurmountable. Layoffs, cutbacks, and internal battle cries of short staffing make your banner for customer relations a perfect target. Keeping the customer relations banner flying isn't easy when all you seem to be doing is making more demands on people or when your nose is buried in reports, requests, and memos. Keeping customer relations excellence going isn't easy. It takes courageous people to get the job done and to keep at it—forever.

☐ Final Suggestions

As you make and remake decisions about staffing your strategy for service excellence, you must beware of these traps:

- *"The patient representative can handle it."* Hundreds of hospitals have assigned the responsibility for customer relations leadership to a person or people who already carry endless responsibility: the training professional, the patient representative, the director of volunteers. More often than not, the patient representative spearheads customer relations and is intent on seeing the organization develop a far-reaching strategy. These people are "awarded" customer relations as an additional responsibility but get no additional staff and no decrease in their other responsibilities. This situation is not just unfair; it's usually unworkable and leads to an impossible bind for the person involved. Placing the responsibility for customer relations in the capable hands of your patient representatives is fine, but make sure that they have adequate support so that they can effectively wear their multiple hats simultaneously.

- *"It's not my job."* On the one hand, you need a director who holds together your customer relations strategy and nurtures the other people involved. On the other hand, once you name a person as the one responsible for customer relations, others in the organization may sigh with relief that the customer relations responsibility is now taken care of. Somehow, your higher-ups must make it clear that customer relations is everybody's job and that every manager and supervisor at every level is expected to make bold moves for improved customer relations.

- *"You can handle it alone. I'm sure of it."* So often, one person is assigned the customer relations responsibility and is given no support staff. The customer relations coordinator must have clerical support and a squad of people somewhere in the organization to help steer a sound course.

- *"I trust you to run with it. Now don't bother me with it."* Delegation to a fault, that's what this sentiment reflects. Some administrators delegate customer relations responsibility to a hyperresponsible person in the organization and hope and expect that the administrative team can thus avoid being bothered with it. When the coordinator approaches them for help, authority, resources, and the like, the higher-ups make the director feel inadequate to the task. Service excellence needs to be a pervasive systemwide priority. A coordinator can manage the strategy but cannot be expected to make it all happen without substantial administrative support.

- *Short-sighted screening for the job.* Sometimes, the enthusiast gets the job; but perhaps this enthusiast isn't the right person for the job. Even an enthusiast can lack the mix of skills (leadership, energy, organizational ability, and an obsession for detail) to accomplish the job efficiently and effectively. Make sure that your key people have the mix of energy, credibility, and skill needed to carry out their mandate effectively.

- *Out on a limb, alone.* The mover-and-shaker coordinator is frequently left stranded with an enormous responsibility, perhaps in a one-person department without a strong bond to a mover-and-shaker administrator who pulls strings for them. The isolation that results for these people is intense and diminishes their ability to do their jobs. Administration needs to position the customer relations coordinator in a place that reflects its priority on service excellence and links the coordinator to the powers that be.

- *"It's not that hard."* Most administrators could not do the job of the customer relations coordinator. It takes a degree of stamina, creativity, people management, and diverse skills. Customer relations coordinators need support, and yet they are frequently denied access to professional conferences with peers, money for subscribing to newsletters, and other forms of support for their growing profession.

- *"Customer relations and patient representation are the same."* Hospitals need patient representatives, who serve as advocates and change agents. They also need physician and employee representatives. Patient representatives help patients, physicians, and employees navigate the system and get their needs met. Along the way, they play a major role in catching, tracking, and responding to complaints. The job of the customer relations coordinator is not identical to the job of the patient representative. One key role of the coordinator's job is to institute a multistep change strategy that primarily involves interactions with employees and doctors. The coordinator's job is heavily administrative, involving strategy implementation and long-range project management. A hospital that chooses to get along without a patient representative is missing a key function that any health care organization that really cares about its patients would not do without. And this function can definitely not be replaced by a coordinator of a customer relations strategy. If it is, then the administrators' understanding of customer relations has gone berserk. In sum, your organization needs both roles and adequate staffing to accomplish both roles well.

Every customer group needs someone in your organization to be its special advocate. That is why so many hospitals have patient representatives, physician relations people, and employee relations people; and these roles are all essential. However, if your organization wants to perpetuate an organizationwide, far-reaching strategy for service excellence, it must have one person or a team of persons who can spearhead, oversee, and prod this complex and comprehensive strategy for the long-term benefit of the entire organization and those the organization serves.

Resistance to a Strategy for Service Excellence

Resistance to strategies for service excellence is inevitable even in the best of organizations, because striving for excellence requires change and change breeds resistance. Gail Scott, director of service excellence services at the Einstein Consulting Group and an expert resistance-handler says, "The challenge is to prevent staff resistance through the development of carefully wrought motivational strategies and to confront directly the resistance that erupts despite best efforts at prevention. Ignoring or denying resistance does not make it go away."

Resistance can take many forms, as seen in the following examples:

- A superior gives lip service to the concept of service excellence. He's a hard-line manager who lives by "do as I say, not as I do." He expects his people to conform to rules with no training or staff development.
- Helene always has an excuse. The other patient, the other tech, the other department is always the cause of whatever problem is at hand. She has a victim personality and is quick to point the finger at everyone but herself. She reacts the same way with regard to service excellence. She's exemplary, she thinks. The other people cause the problem.
- Mark works as a nurse, but you'd think he complained for a living. He is always annoyed, always griping, and always lowering the

morale of his colleagues. He is quick to say: "This will never work; we're too short-staffed" and "administration doesn't care anyway." The glass is always half-empty, never half-full. Mark sees only the pitfalls in customer relations and the burden of more pressure to perform.

- What does Leslie think about service excellence? You can't be sure. She's late for task force meetings. She sits quietly with raised eyebrows. She always has an excuse for why she didn't do what she promised to do.
- Wanda keeps you wondering. Sometimes she seems to be an enthusiast and sometimes the barrier to action. She is inconsistent and reacts without thinking.
- Sandy still feels insulted by the concept of service excellence no matter what you do or say. She's seen herself as a superstar for years.
- Larry works in engineering. He doesn't see the point of involving everybody in customer relations because he doesn't serve patients and he's busy.
- Your whole emphasis on service excellence passes Mary by. She thinks your hospital is fine the way it is, especially compared with other hospitals. She also thinks that courtesy is learned in childhood. If an employee is rude now, she thinks you can't change them.
- Lou is a department head. He's noncommittal about customer relations, neither enthusiastic nor unenthusiastic. Satisfied with the status quo, he does just enough to get by when it comes to customer relations. An inspiration, he isn't. Excellence among his people is not expected.

However, before examining methods of preventing or minimizing all of these and more kinds of resistance, consider that resistance to service excellence is normal. The normal response to any kind of change is resistance. Behavioral scientist Kurt Lewin described organizational change as a three-step sequential process:

- Step 1: Unfreezing or thawing out established patterns
- Step 2: Changing or moving to a new pattern
- Step 3: Refreezing or maintaining the new pattern

Resistance is especially inherent in the first step, unfreezing. Unfreezing is inevitably unsettling, because it stems from tension that drives people to search for new ways to do things. Such tension is typically generated by an awareness of competitive pressures, falling standards, image problems, a financial downturn, and the like. If your people don't feel this tension, you have to take explicit steps to create mild states of anxiety, or your people will not be motivated to change.

No wonder the concept of service excellence meets resistance. Who wants to feel anxiety and pressure to abandon old ways that may have worked fine for years?

□ The Most Frequent Types of Resisters

Although resistance takes many forms, employees who resist the concept of service excellence tend to fall largely into three groups. Some persons are insulted by the notion of a strategy for service excellence. They already think of themselves as professional when it comes to extending themselves to patients. Other persons are cynics who doubt the effectiveness of or their organization's long-term commitment to service excellence: "this is just another flash-in-the-pan," or "you must be joking, you can't change people." Finally, other persons are so full of resentment toward the organization that they refuse to cooperate. They will only get better when they are treated better by the organization: "If you muckamucks give me the respect I deserve and solve the problems that make my life miserable, then I'll bend over backward for our patients; but until then, get off my back!"

The insulted are insulted for a reason. The cynics are cynical for a reason. The resentful are resentful for a reason. Arguing against their reasons or attempting to squelch them doesn't help. Their reasons are real and contain at least a grain of truth. Still, you have to be so committed to your vision of service excellence that you don't allow these reasons to put you off course. After all, what reasons justify lowering the standards of excellence or not expecting high standards from employees?

The bottom line is:

> Resistance is inevitable.
> You will never eliminate it entirely.
> *But you can't let it rule.*

So, what can you do? The following suggestions may help:

- Come to terms with your commitment to service excellence and customer relations. Decide firmly what you really want to achieve until your vision is unflinching. Hang on to your vision despite bouts with resistance. Don't permit yourself to lose your balance.
- You know your employees and physicians. Anticipate the forms of resistance that are likely to emerge.
- Plan and prepare your strategy with potential pockets of resistance in mind. Consciously build in rationales and approaches designed

to minimize the anticipated resistance instead of fueling it.
- No matter how hard you try, you can't prevent all resistance, so prepare to react skillfully when it rears its frustrating head.

Drawing on the wisdom of top sales people, here are tips for selling your colleagues on your plans for service excellence:

- Anticipate the most likely objections to your strategy for service excellence: Take the other person's point of view. Imagine the worst possible response. Ask friends to help you anticipate. And don't worry, the responses won't really be as bad as you anticipate.
- Presell the benefits. Make a list of the objections you may be able to eliminate if you can convince your employees of the value of your request, plan, or opportunity.
- Work these benefits and proofs into your approach. Emphasize them. Address potential resistance even before anyone voices it.
- Set up a strategy so you'll be able to handle objections not easily eliminated in your approach. Leave time to handle objections. Take them seriously. Respond if you can.

You can't expect to anticipate every objection that a colleague may voice. However, you can generate greater cooperation if you take a little time to plan for objections.

□ An Ounce of Prevention

Taking measures to prevent resistance is more efficient than trying to cure it. You can prevent resistance by:

- Encouraging employee participation
- Paying attention to the feelings and concerns of employees
- Developing exquisitely clear performance expectations and putting "teeth" into the performance evaluation process
- Providing assertive and inspiring leadership
- Keeping your promises

Encouraging Employee Participation

A basic tool of prevention is to involve a wide range of employees who are informal opinion leaders in your organization in the needs assessment and planning for service excellence. Any diverse group of opinion leaders tends to include potential malcontents. Here are the steps for working with the malcontents:

- Directly and constructively solicit their criticism and use it in forming strategies for service excellence. No institution is perfect, and employee complaints are usually at least partially legitimate. Redressing complaints about, for example, equipment or cumbersome procedures, often enables employees to deliver better service to customers of the hospital.
- Solicit people's advice about strategy questions. Such action causes potential resisters to have an investment or stake in the eventual strategy.
- By involving a wide variety of people up front, you are inviting them to bring their feelings out in the open where you can handle them. If you let these feelings stay hidden, they'll eat away at and erode your best efforts later.

Involving employees in the strategy for service excellence shows them that their concerns and advice are appreciated and increases their self-esteem. These feelings reinforce their positive feelings about your organization and weaken their resistance to your strategy for service excellence.

Paying Attention to Feelings of Employees

Once again, the three groups most likely to show resistance are the insulted, the cynical, and the resentful.

- *The insulted.* Acknowledge that people are already good at customer relations but that being "good" isn't good enough in today's environment. Then concentrate your efforts on raising awareness, not on training, and emphasize moving from "good" to "great." This action sends a motivating, nonpunitive message. Emphasize the new economic challenges hospitals face and the need "to pull out all the stops" to compete effectively. Tell the truth and avoid rhetoric. Workshops shouldn't be pep talks. Employees need to know that service excellence and customer relations aren't grounded in lofty rhetoric but are competitive responses to the increasingly fierce health care market. When employees see the organization relying on them to be the "excellence factor," customer relations is flattering, not insulting.
- *The cynics.* Donald Kanter and Philip Mirvis of Boston University find an "us against them" syndrome surfacing in the United States. They claim that handling hostile, cynical staff members who have a high opinion of themselves is becoming a central problem in managing, let alone in creating, change in our human resources.
  The new generation of cynics requires thoughtful approaches to

corporate culture and therefore to customer relations. According to Kanter and Mirvis in "Managing Jaundiced Workers" (*New Management*, 1986 Spring, 3[4]:50-54), cynics believe that corporate communications are designed to deceive and manipulate them. They suggest that communicating with cynics requires a special approach with these features:

—When presenting information, allow all sides to be heard. Even antimanagement positions should be heard so that cynics cannot claim a cover-up.

—Communications should be phrased so that people have a chance to make up their own minds and should not be simply direct transmissions of management policy.

—Communications should not raise workers' expectations unduly.

—Management presentations should be factual and cool. Information, not propaganda, should be offered.

—Communications should come from members of senior management who are known to the work force.

—If the message is important, its initial presentation should be followed up by informal, small-group meetings at which the message is reinforced and fence-sitters are encouraged to consider all sides.

Confronted with your strategy for service excellence, cynics become skeptical. Perhaps they had embraced similar programs in the past, only to see them fade away because of waning administrative support or lack of follow up. The cynics need to know that this program isn't just another flash in the pan. Workshops should emphasize that the administration has made a serious, ongoing commitment to service excellence and that a long-term plan is in place. If the cynics walk out of a workshop expecting no results, they'll put forth no effort and thus be proved right. Challenge them to suspend their disbelief. Dare them to excel, and convince them that their efforts will be continuously augmented by the entire organization.

- *The resentful.* Develop with executive management a clearly defined mechanism for employee participation in problem identification and problem solving, for prompt action on employee suggestions, and for prompt feedback so that employees know the results of their complaints, whether or not they are actually resolved. Resentful employees need to be aware that your organization recognizes the need for extensive, ongoing "body work," and not just a glossy "paint job" in terms of customer relations.

Good faith has to be developed between the administration and employees who resent it. Workshops can help by offering employees the chance to vent their frustrations, frustrations that should be seriously listened to, recorded, and turned over to the right people for action. All complaints deserve a response. If changes are made, tell employees. If changes can't be made, tell them why. Preventing resentment requires dialogue.

Ideally, these resistance-prevention approaches should be implemented at the beginning of a strategy for service excellence. However, these same techniques can be introduced at any point in an ongoing program to curb existing resistance.

Developing Exquisitely Clear Performance Expectations

Ambiguity about job-performance expectations breeds limit-testing on the part of a small but visible number of employees. The antidote is clarity, unequivocal and explicit customer relations expectations backed up by enforced consequences for an employee's actions. As the discussion of accountability in chapter 6 explains, your organization needs to put "teeth" into your customer relations expectations, and make the "teeth" known to your employees before you enforce them so that they have a chance to choose to perform.

Providing Assertive and Inspiring Leadership

Eliminate double standards because double standards often breed resistance. One of the most effective ways to soften resistance is through positive role modeling by executives and middle managers. Managers must form excellent customer relations habits that they exhibit visibly as they interact with hospital employees. When resistant employees see this behavior, they feel much less righteous in their resistance. When they do not see managers practicing what they preach, the seeds of resistance blossom.

☐ Minimizing Resistance

To repeat, you can minimize resistance, but you can't entirely prevent it no matter how cleverly or meticulously you anticipate it. However, these three response techniques can help you to minimize existing resistance:

- See resistance as feedback and listen to it.
- Enforce expectations, resistance or no resistance.
- Develop a repertoire of resistance comebacks.

See Resistance as Feedback

First of all, don't keel over or get angry when resistance strikes. Adjust your mind set so that you see resistance as feedback and as useful feedback at that. Listen to it; let it help you develop your ongoing strategy. Act on it if you find it worthwhile.

When asked questions you can't answer, admit it. If you fudge, the resister sees your pretense and loses trust in you. Better to say, "That's a good question; let me think about it" or "That's a tough question; let me see if I can get an answer for you." Then regain the initiative by asking, for example, how detailed an answer the resister thinks is necessary, how soon the resister wants an answer, and so forth. Take notes on everything the person says to show that you're taking the questions seriously and, in fact, are already working on it.

Enforce Expectations

Hold people accountable no matter what. Some people resist or rebel in hopes of being let off the hook. If their resistance reaps these benefits for them, expect an epidemic of resistance.

An employee who does not meet your standards for service excellence cannot be allowed to get by. You put "teeth" in your customer relations by developing policies, job-description statements, behavioral expectations, a performance appraisal system, and the like. Now, you must follow through. Without enforcement, excellence crumbles; and the same few people who drag down morale and the image of the organization continue to do so, dragging good people down with them.

Performance deficiency must be clearly communicated. Frank counseling or disciplinary interviews should point out unacceptable behavior and suggest specific alternative behaviors. A supervisor has a responsibility to be candid and assertive. To avoid confrontation or to be taken in by alibis is to cop out.

Definite and standardized consequences should be in place to support performance expectations. Written performance reviews should reflect if performance has been poor. Raises should not be automatic, but contingent on merit. Equally rewarding bad employees and good ones undermines incentive, morale, and ultimately, the entire drive for service excellence. The final consequence for the resistant worker is dismissal. Firing an employee is something no manager likes to do, but tolerating poor or even mediocre performance compromises your entire commitment to service excellence. As with any disciplinary action, the reasons for firing an employee should be fully documented.

Here's a case study that demonstrates how to bring a mediocre employee up to service excellence standards and points out specific techniques to use with problem employees. Debbie had been the receptionist for the x-ray department for seven years. During that time, the hospital made a series of budget cutbacks that increased her work load. More recently, the hospital had instituted a customer relations program. The problem is that Debbie was not performing her role as a welcomer at all well. Rather than setting people's minds at ease at the start of their visits, her curt conduct and generally caustic manner offended patients and their families and gave them a distasteful overall impression of the hospital. Debbie, who expressed resentment about her increased paperwork and seemed to consider welcoming duties an annoying interruption, dismissed the hospital-wide emphasis on hospitality stressed by the customer relations program. Frank, Debbie's manager, had been aware of the situation for some time, but he simply overlooked it to avoid a confrontation. The problem came to a head when two x-ray technicians complained that by the time patients got to them, they were not only apprehensive about having X rays but were also irritated and defensive because of Debbie's gruff behavior. Finally, Frank decided he had to act.

The first step wasn't to meet with Debbie, but rather to plan a meeting. Frank wrote a list of specific behavioral shortcomings in Debbie's typical greeting of a patient. The list included her habit of making the patient wait before looking up from her paperwork, then giving a what-do-you-want-can't-you-see-I'm busy facial expression, throwing down her pen, and either forcing the patient to speak first or gruffly asking what the patient wanted.

Frank then wrote down how these behaviors had a negative impact on the hospital. This step may seem unnecessary, but writing out answers to probable objections is helpful when it comes to fielding them in tense meetings and also helps the manager to decide which behaviors are most important to insist upon. If a manager can't justify the importance of a certain behavior, it's probably not crucial to the customer relations effort. Frank also quickly sketched a picture of the fiercely competitive health care marketplace and the importance of outstanding customer relations.

Finally, Frank enumerated in specific behavioral terms the standards he expected Debbie to uphold. These standards included setting aside any other work and quickly serving the arriving patients, taking the initiative by making eye contact and speaking first, offering a pleasant greeting and introducing herself by name, and so forth.

This planning stage is probably the most important part of approaching the problem employee. Unfortunately, most managers make the mistake of omitting it. When you get face-to-face with an

281

antagonistic employee who sees such a meeting as an adversarial situation, be prepared to identify specific problems and specific solutions. Before going one-on-one, anticipate objections so that your replies are well thought out and not impromptu. Not surprisingly, problem employees don't tend to thank you for your feedback when you confront them. Instead, they try to put you on the spot. Unless you're prepared to stand firm and assert your bottom-line expectations and unless you're convinced of the validity of these expectations, you're likely to lose control of the meeting and say things that will then commit you to accept lowered standards.

Within a week of deciding to act, Frank met with Debbie. Because this meeting was not a disciplinary one, Frank was careful to use a positive tone and to make his presentation in a problem-solution format rather than to seem to be reprimanding her. Throughout the meeting, he was responsive without backing down.

Debbie's first objection was that she was overworked. Frank acknowledged that her work load was heavy but explained how that could not excuse rudeness or be allowed to justify poor customer relations. He explained that her customer relations responsibilities were not an addition to her work but part of it, and he clearly set those responsibilities as her top priority.

When Debbie argued that her work style had not changed and that to suddenly throw these new expectations at her was unfair, Frank candidly admitted that he should have approached her before. Never having done so was his mistake, but that was not reason enough to tolerate inadequate performance in the future.

Debbie asked what would happen if she didn't go along with these new expectations. Frank stated that if she refused to meet the performance standards of the hospital, she would be subject, like anyone else, to its disciplinary process.

In this case, Debbie eventually saw that Frank's expectations were not negotiable. She finally accepted the fact that continued customer relations problems would result in disciplinary action in the short run and dismissal in the long run. She may have continued to *feel* resistant, but she took steps to behave appropriately anyway. The point is that clear, enforced expectations that are *not* negotiable are vital. They stamp out resistance that's used to manipulate managers into lowering their expectations.

Resistance Comebacks

What about those annoying one-liners that catch you off guard in the hallways and elevators?

- "How's your sweet little customer relations program going?"
- "Marge, you're not smiling!"
- "Customer relations—the farce of the year. When's the next showing?"
- "Don't tell me we're going to have to schedule our people again for charm school!"
- "How did a sharp person like you get suckered into this customer relations bit?"

The resistance expert at the Einstein Consulting Group, Gail Scott, has developed a tool kit of 16 skills for responding to sarcastic cracks, loaded innuendoes, or straightforward resistant comments:

- *Be a sounding board.* Find out why. Ask open-ended questions. Let employees vent their frustrations. Express concern and empathy.
- *Enlist support.* Don't be afraid to ask for help. Be clear about your own identification with the service excellence mission.
- *Stand firm.* Let resisters know that customer relations goes with the territory. Keep emphasizing that customer relations is everyone's job.
- *Show humor.* "What have we got to lose?" "Why not try it; things can't get much worse." "We'll show them all."
- *Share benefits.* Point out to the resisters what's in it for them. Give good logical reasons why customer relations is really good for employees: for example, less stress and a more pleasant, cooperative environment.
- *Meet resisters halfway.* Rearrange schedules. Solve problems. Offer alternatives. Use their input.
- *Charm and disarm.* Make resisters feel special. Let them see that they are good and are valued but that, of course, everyone "has room for fine tuning."
- *Tell a tale.* Sometimes, people need to hear other people's customer relations success stories.
- *Command respect.* Don't let any abusive resistance out there anger you. Remind the abusive resister that you're a person, not a thing.
- *Give logical explanations.* Describe why customer relations is good for the hospital, for patients, and for the resisters to the strategy. Share the realities of the economic picture. Point to competition, market research, and so forth.
- *Switch the focus.* Ask the resisters questions. Put them on the defensive. Weaken their arguments.
- *Change the environment.* Surprise resisters. Make quick improvement so they see that something is actually happening.

- *Get their opinions.* Engage resisters as opinion leaders. Involve them in think tanks, focus groups, and advisory committees.
- *Hold up a mirror.* Show resisters how their resistance sounds and what it looks like. Some people don't even know they're being negative.
- *Provide an experience.* Let the resisters talk to patients and view a positive interaction. A good role model helps.
- *Take a strong personal stand.* Stick your neck out if you believe in what you're doing: "You might think I'm crazy, but I don't. I really believe that customer relations is going to be good for us, and I'm going to do what I can to make it work."

□ Final Suggestions

Resistance to the changes that are required if your organization is to more toward excellent service is inevitable. As you encounter this resistance, consider these final suggestions:

- *Don't label resisters as negative.* Resistance is an expected stage in change, and therefore you should read resistance as progress in making people aware of new, more ambitious expectations. Then, with empathy, help them grieve over the past so that they can move forward.
- *Don't harbor grudges against resisters.* So often, people spearheading strategies for service excellence have turned initially resistant people into believers and supporters. Remember the power of your own expectations and *expect* resisters to become your strategy's success stories and best advocates.

Resistance to change is more than just inevitable; it's also a natural reaction to often unsettling changes in the status quo. Remember that everyone, even the most forward-thinking individual, has some difficulty handling changes in the status quo. Consequently, resistance to change is a force that must be planned for as you develop your strategy for service excellence and a source of energy that you can use to build eventual support for that strategy. Because resistance is natural, expect it and don't be intimidated by it.

Service Excellence in Special Settings

A generic recipe for successful service excellence doesn't exist. The customer relations strategist must consider the differences between teaching hospitals and community hospitals, emergency departments and physicians' offices, pediatric settings and nursing homes, and other special settings when evolving a strategy for service excellence.

This chapter highlights unique characteristics of 13 specific settings that deserve special attention in planning an ongoing strategy for service excellence:

- Teaching hospitals
- Denominational organizations
- Public hospitals
- Pediatric hospitals
- Psychiatric settings
- Unionized settings
- Ambulatory care settings
- Rehabilitation hospitals
- Chronic care settings
- Nursing homes
- Emergency departments
- Rural hospitals
- Multicultural settings

The problem with a chapter like this is that stereotypes and overgeneralizations are inevitable. This book could overlook the subject for fear of overgeneralizing, or the issues typical of special settings can be discussed with up-front apologies for offending people because of generalizations. The latter option has been chosen because it may help the reader learn from the experience of others at relatively similar institutions.

☐ Teaching Hospitals

Teaching hospitals are unique in many ways, but nine specifics relate to customer relations excellence.

- *Large organizations with competing missions.* Teaching hospitals tend to be relatively large, with three powerful and often competing objectives: teaching, research, and patient care. Depending on whom you ask, these three objectives vary in importance. Although the three objectives do not have to conflict, many insiders do report considerable conflict. For instance, university researchers may be focused on developing new knowledge and so may show relative disinterest in diagnosis, which is important to the patient. Researchers usually only have a stake in patient care if it conforms to their research needs. The teaching faculty, on the other hand, may be more interested in what residents and interns can learn from specific cases and so may overlook the patient as person. Meanwhile, the people most concerned about patient care gnash their teeth when they see teaching and research activities interfere with what the patient needs.

   The implications for service excellence in teaching hospitals are not simple. The leadership in the teaching hospital must crystallize its vision for customer relations and communicate the fit between its vision and the priorities of the hospital. Also, the customer relations strategist needs to develop rationales for the priority on service excellence that respond to the top priority of each segment of the hospital environment. What's best for research and teaching may conflict with the patient's best interest. In a teaching hospital, everyone needs to bend over backward to respect the dignity of the patient. After all, reams of students will examine and reexamine the patient, ask the same questions over and over, request tests, and be replaced tomorrow by a different, uninformed, recycled student. The service excellence mind set can be a problem in this kind of environment and therefore needs all the more powerful initial propulsion by hospital leadership in the teaching hospital environment.

- *High tech.* Frequently the hotbed of state-of-the-art medical equipment and technique, teaching hospitals tend to attract staff and physicians who themselves are attracted to technological sophistication. Some say that high tech mitigates against high touch. The polarity between high tech and high touch needs to be confronted as part of the strategy for service excellence.
- *The status hierarchy.* Although all hospitals seem to have a defined pecking order, teaching hospitals have even bigger gaps between the superdoctors at the top and the housekeepers at the bottom. This status differential aggravates interpersonal problems and resentments among employees and doctors and promotes an atmosphere of disrespect and indignity.

  The implications for customer relations are that status issues have to be confronted. Otherwise, employees at the bottom of the status hierarchy are infuriated by the obvious double standard that the leadership fosters. Also, your strategy should include intergroup team building so that the different status layers begin to get an understanding of one another's daily experiences and frustrations. Finally, you need to pay special attention to employee recognition, particularly methods for recognizing the critical contributions of the lower-status people in an environment in which the superspecialist doctors and the research gurus with power, prestige, bonuses, and perks are usually the ones elevated and spotlighted by administrators.
- *Who's in charge?* Most teaching hospitals have a convoluted governance structure and thus inherent conflicts between university administrators and hospital administrators who each have rules and policies. Also to be considered are the governing structures among the doctors. When people want to initiate a strategy, they frequently don't even know who has the power to approve or commit resources. By the time all the key parties have input into new program thrusts, years can pass. The result is incredibly slow decision making and even paralysis, which causes extreme frustration among the people trying to advance a seedling strategy for service excellence. Take personnel practices, for example. Do the university's personnel practices govern hospital staff, or does the hospital have its own practices? Can the hospital develop employee expectations that are much more stringent than are those that the university develops for nonhospital employees? How about the people who spend part of their time in each of the two environments? Customer relations strategists need to thoroughly understand the structure of the hospital, especially who makes decisions, so that time is not wasted going to the wrong people for decisions.

287

- *Doctors at all stages.* The structure of the medical staff is a complex of layers and relationships. Medical students rotate through various services every six weeks, and residents provide intense patient care during what can be inhuman 20-hour days for low pay. Also part of the complex mix are salaried physicians with a stake in the organization and attending physicians who threaten to switch hospitals if their status and ease of practice don't get better. The multiple segments of the medical staff in teaching hospitals means that involving doctors in customer relations strategies is difficult. However, the doctors obviously must be part of the solution. All doctors can't be lumped together and treated similarly. To advance customer relations, a different strategy that takes into consideration politics, history, degree of involvement, and commitment to the organization usually needs to be developed for each layer. Every layer also needs to be involved in planning the nature of involvement for that layer.

- *For the hospital or the whole university?* A clear decision must be made up front about whether the strategy for service excellence is for the hospital only or also for the university. In some cases, people have started with the hospital and treated service excellence there separately. Then, after making headway and gaining optimism about the power of an explicit strategy, the university side is targeted for an equally far-reaching service excellence effort. Interestingly, universities, like hospitals, have entered a hotly competitive era and their dynamics are similar. Status differences exist between the sacred tenured faculty and the rest of the staff; governance is confusing because of faculty-administration conflicts (like doctor-administration conflicts in hospitals), and organizational practices have frequently been developed for the convenience of the faculty instead of the students (like hospital practices being developed for the convenience of the provider and health care professionals instead of the patient). The point is that the surprisingly similar dynamics between hospitals and universities mean that transferring a successful strategy for service excellence from the hospital to the university is not difficult.

- *A web of systems problems.* Given a triple mission, high-tech care, and layers of rotating care givers, teaching hospitals suffer from a web of interlocking and sometimes strangulating systems problems that interfere with employee customer relations and patient satisfaction. Examples of systems problems include scheduling, lack of continuity from one care giver to another, missing charts, duplicate testing, student after student asking the patient the same questions over and over, slow turnaround time on lab results, fragmented discharge planning, and transportation problems.

Strategies for service excellence cannot ignore these problems because they have such a powerful effect on the ability of care givers to extend themselves to patients and doctors. When systems problems frustrate, tempers flare, patients wait, people point fingers at one another, and a soothing, compassionate atmosphere is fantasy. As part of your plan for service excellence, you must incorporate a system for identifying and attacking once and for all systems problems that impede excellent customer relations, especially in teaching hospitals.

- *Student involvement a must.* Residents, interns, and rotators (students who spend short stints in several areas) provide most of the patient care in teaching hospitals. Yet, these people tend to be transient, overworked, and uncommitted to your hospital. Consequently, your customer relations strategy must involve these groups, or you will not see significant changes happen. These groups are too important, too potentially helpful, and too potentially hurtful to your strategy for service excellence.

- *Sicker people, hyperstress environment, burned-out staff.* Because high-tech hospitals tend to attract the sicker people and the more complex illnesses, the environment is especially stressful for the people who do the work. The work is draining, as staff witness personal tragedies and miracles. Some staff insulate or harden themselves in self-defense. Others crumble and leave from the onslaught of emotion. To advance service excellence, you need to pay attention to the care givers' emotions and needs for compassionate, attentive, and supportive behavior toward one another. To focus only on service excellence toward the patient in these environments denies the reality of the care givers' experience. Also, your strategy for service excellence needs to include programs that help employees with stress and burnout.

☐ Denominational or Church-Related Settings

Typically, denominational or church-related settings already have a strong mission and set of values that drive the organization and its people. Service excellence and the language used to describe the strategy need to be expressed in light of these values and not as a thing apart. For example, if the hospital has a mission statement that includes dignity as one of its five values, the word *dignity* could be used repeatedly as part of the strategy's rhetoric. The more the customer relations approach fits and enhances the existing mission, the more likely that customer relations is a long-term, more explicit theme in the hospital's culture.

Sometimes strategies for service excellence draw on economic arguments, such as competition, declining admissions, or the aggressive advertising campaign by the hospital down the street, as the compelling reasons for paying strategic attention to customer relations in a competitive environment. People in denominational settings have to be especially careful to emphasize the altruistic reasons for service excellence; economics should not be the exclusive force behind their actions. Care givers who are working in these settings for spiritual reasons become cynical when only economic arguments are used to justify service excellence and customer relations. Instead, the ideas of "giving," "service," "emotional generosity," and "concern for humanity" must be acknowledged and reinforced.

People in these settings feel that customer relations is nothing new. For them, the more important focus is on moving from good to excellent and from inconsistent to consistent so that every patient gets the quality of compassionate care that the hospital prides itself on.

☐ Public Hospitals

Public hospitals typically serve sicker and poorer people. On top of that, not only are they usually underfunded, but many are governed by politicians rather than health care professionals. City councils, county seats, and state bodies determine their fate and funding. Also, the employees in many such hospitals are under Civil Service, which places severe constraints on hiring and personnel practices. For some hospitals, getting rid of incompetent people is next to impossible because of stringent Civil Service guidelines and political ramifications. Some public hospitals are even filled with patronage appointees who are ill-equipped to do the job. However, because public hospitals serve the poor, they have many dedicated employees who are there to help the poor, employees who know full well that the poor tend to get the short end of the health care stick no matter where they turn.

Because most public hospitals are also teaching hospitals, you can apply all the customer relations implications described earlier for teaching hospitals. Then, because public hospitals are more likely than private hospitals to be unionized, add the complexities that unionization involves (the issue of unionization is discussed later in this chapter).

On top of everything else, you must confront the low organizationwide self-esteem of many public hospitals. Ironically, because public hospitals serve the indigent, the community usually looks down on the hospital compared with private hospitals that attract insured patients. Employees, then, internalize the second-class status of the hospital, believing it applies to them as well. This situation can lead to an organizationwide inferiority complex.

Your strategy for service excellence must confront this inferiority complex directly and make it work for service excellence. Consider these words that the Einstein Consulting Group has used to build a commitment for service excellence among public hospital employees:

> Why is customer relations being emphasized here? We refuse to buy into the second-class status that some people attribute to us. We are going to outdistance the competition in service for the poor, the people who most deserve the best this society can give. We are thought of as second class because we serve citizens whom the society labels as second class. I ask you, is that right? Have we not bought into this attitude and started to believe that we're second class because the community treats us that way, just because we serve the poor? Shouldn't we feel proud of ourselves for doing this? We must hold our heads high and improve our own self-image. We are sorely needed in this community. And we are good. We want to make our customer relations and patient satisfaction unsurpassed for the sake of our self-image and for the sake of our patients who already get the shaft from society. Through our own behavior, we can work against a fast-developing two-tiered health care system in our own organization. Through attention to stronger customer relations, we have the chance to provide really first-class service and care to the people defined by society as second-class citizens. The result is better health for people who need every chance they can get and higher self-esteem on our parts. Eleanor Roosevelt said, "No one can make you feel inferior without your consent."

The other rationale for customer relations that speaks to most public hospital employees has to do with the need to build public confidence. Through impressive customer relations, employees can alter and improve the image the public has of their institution.

☐ Pediatric Settings

In children's hospitals, the customer is typically the family, not just the child. Family cannot be treated as intruders and interruptions. Families experience a mix of love, fear, worry, helplessness, inadequacy, concern, panic, and sometimes guilt. They are protective and watchful because they have turned their beloved child over to this big hospital for care. No wonder they scrutinize every move anyone makes. No wonder they themselves crave comfort, involvement, and information. No wonder they can be demanding. Your strategy for service excellence needs to emphasize the family as customer and develop ways that staff can make the most of the family's and the child's experiences.

Your strategy should also build mutual support among staff. Staff are intensely involved with the kids. Working with children is, to say the least, emotionally draining. Staff struggle with emotional attachments to the child and family that they know are likely to be fleeting. Employees need help in coping with these emotions, handling stress, and renewing their professional resources. Within your strategy for service excellence, consider providing experiences in which staff can share emotions and rejuvenate their ability to extend themselves to children and families. The slightest focus on "cosmetic" or superficial customer relations in an atmosphere so fraught with pain and feeling is doomed to be disappointing.

Behaviors particularly important in pediatric settings include:

- Explaining things thoroughly in terms both kids and family can grasp
- Believing that there's no such thing as too many questions or dumb questions
- Treating parents with respect and avoiding judgmental attitudes and behaviors about the way they treat their children

Amenities especially are critically important in children's hospitals. Can parents stay overnight? Can they stay close to their child while the child is in surgery? Are the colors cheerful? Does the unit have things for the children to do, distractions? Have people taken special steps to demystify intimidating machinery by giving it names like Herman or Zelda?

Generally, the staff in children's hospitals are supremely people oriented. Therefore, the emphasis in your strategy for service excellence should be on consistent excellence toward every type of customer and on building supportive, nourishing bonds among staff.

☐ Psychiatric Settings

The first person who has the nerve to suggest the need for customer relations in a psychiatric setting should receive accolades. Professionals are likely to respond as did one anonymous psychiatrist: "How dare you tell me how to behave toward patients! I am an expert on human behavior."

Psychiatric settings are staffed by professionals who specialize in psychoemotional health and behavior, which includes interpersonal behavior. Consequently, many may be offended at a hint that their organization needs an explicit customer relations strategy. To succeed, then, strategists need to become quite articulate about what customer relations means in this setting and what it does not mean. Staff expertise about human behavior must be acknowledged, but behaviors that interfere with patient and family satisfaction must also be confronted.

If your customer relations message insists that "the customer is always right," it will be met with understandably vehement resistance. Understandably, psychiatric professionals claim that patients in a psychiatric setting should not be catered to but instead should be encouraged to do everything possible for themselves. Also, the responsible professional believes in expressing frustration, impatience, and anger at the patient if this response is realistic in light of the patient's behavior. The same situation applies to the patient's family. The challenge is to extend excellent customer relations when appropriate but, at the same time, to do nothing to interfere with clinical judgments about what patients need. The "pampering" that may be appropriate in an acute care hospital setting must be questioned in terms of each patient's treatment objectives.

What Behaviors Then?

Behaviors that are important to emphasize include being consistently courteous toward patients, making eye contact, calling people by name, and saying hello. Even drugged patients are aware of what's happening. Other key behaviors include treating patients as adults, taking pains to protect their dignity, explaining what you're doing in plain language to both patient and family, describing your approaches, and inviting questions and discussion.

Also, consider professional dress. Many people feel that dress standards should distinguish patients from staff. Traditionally, psychiatric hospitals have had lenient dress codes that sometimes interfere with the family's confidence in them as health care professionals.

Stigma and the Family's Response

In addition to behavioral issues, the issue of stigma must be considered. Many people feel that a stigma is attached to staff, patients, and families associated with psychiatric settings, and as a result, treating the family as an important customer is even more essential. Staff can help to minimize this stigma by expressing warmth and acceptance toward families and by demonstrating pride in their association with them.

The family members who visit are anxious and often embarrassed. They appreciate the comforts of homey colors and noninstitutional amenities and environments that obliterate the image the public got from the movie *One Flew over the Cuckoo's Nest.* And they talk about their loved one's experiences in the psychiatric setting.

The Impeccable Pecking Order

A rigid pecking order tends to exist in psychiatric settings. This pecking order puts distance between the various professionals: the psychiatrists, the psychologists, recreation therapists, and the dietary workers. Your strategy for service excellence should deliberately jangle this pecking order by confronting its negative consequences, mixing groups, and providing explicit team-building experiences. All people in the psychiatric setting need to communicate and cooperate for the sake of the patient and family.

In terms of building specific skills, in addition to the usual, consider helping staff at all levels cope with violent behavior in appropriate ways. The dynamics involved here are particularly sticky from a customer relations point of view. Staff need and deserve special help, so that the patient, family, and they themselves know that tough situations are handled appropriately and sensitively.

☐ Unionized Settings

The organization's informal opinion leaders, including union representatives and others, should be involved from the start of your strategy for service excellence. Solicit their early help in shaping your strategy. Include union and nonunion employees as workshop facilitators. Make sure you review with union people any new behavioral expectations you are building into personnel policies or any changes you're making in people's job descriptions. The key is to have no surprises.

Generally, union people seem to accept explicit customer relations standards and their integration into personnel practices. The key is to be explicit, write down the expectations, enforce them, and apply them to all people in a consistent, nondiscriminatory way. Actually, all of these points should apply to union and nonunion settings alike because they reflect good sense.

☐ Ambulatory Care Settings

Ambulatory care settings, such as urgicenters, surgicenters, imaging centers, outpatient clinics, occupational health centers, HMOs, community health centers, and physicians' offices, serve patients in the short term, and as a result, care givers have little time to build relationships. Thus, staff may tend to depersonalize interactions because they see some patients so seldom. Why bother to "connect"? Why bother to learn their names? This interaction pattern produces a definite risk that the employee will see the patient as an ailment and not as a complete person. Also, ambulatory care centers tend to emphasize efficiency so that many patients can be seen quickly.

From a customer relations point of view, ambulatory care situations require staff to establish personal relationships with the patient quickly if they are to impress customers and influence the likelihood that customers feel "connected" enough to your setting to use it loyally in the future and say good things about it to family and friends. First and last impressions are especially crucial because not much happens in between. Staff need to take the initiative, to offer help, to not wait to be asked, to be courteous and warm, and to always thank the customer. The following are ways to "break the ice" and exhibit courtesy: introduce yourself (which is rarely done), call the patient by name, explain plainly what you're doing, invite questions and feedback about the patient's understanding of what's happening, explain and ease long waits, provide periodic unsolicited updates about how long the wait will be, and handle bills in a sensitive and confidential manner. Although staff may only have a minute, they can make that minute meaningful and memorable for the patient by exhibiting polished public contact skills. Special training in such skills needs to be a central component in customer relations work in ambulatory care settings.

The special importance of telephone skills should not be forgotten. Unlike hospitals, where doctors make many of the arrangements, customers tend to contact outpatient centers themselves. Therefore, special emphasis must be placed on refining phone interactions with patients.

The importance of other nonpeople factors that have significant customer relations impact should also not be minimized. Take access and convenience, for instance. Parking, clear signs, quick in and out access, convenient transportation, all of these have to work for the good of the patient. Amenities, too, are important. The waiting areas should be comfortable and attractive and have something for patients to do while they wait. Examination rooms should be warm enough. All such amenities are important in ambulatory care settings, because the patient's experience in this setting is usually a limited one.

Amenities, environmental factors, and staff courtesies make a big difference. Your strategy for service excellence then needs to address all of these and their interrelationships. The other implication for customer relations is the need to involve your entire team in your approach.

☐ Rehabilitation Hospitals

Rehabilitation hospitals are unique. Typically, a strong team feeling exists, with physiatrists on staff working closely with other professional and nonprofessional people. The team nature of the effort makes involving physicians in programs with all other employees atypically easy.

As in psychiatric hospitals, the philosophy that the "customer is always right" may conflict with the rehabilitation hospital's treatment goal of independence. When the patient asks, "Can you get me that?" the employee within earshot may appropriately say, "No, you can get it yourself, Jim." Jim may get mad and complain about the lack of service. Your strategy for service excellence should emphasize the importance of *explaining why* you won't do certain things for patients instead of catering to Jim despite his best interest. The employee should also explain this rationale to family members so the push toward independence is not perceived instead as a service inadequacy.

In rehabilitation settings, employees also tend to burn out quickly. Many professionals believe that burnout happens more quickly because of the slowness of the progress many patients are able to make. Lately, employees experience increasing frustration because sicker people are being admitted to their facilities, people with medical complications that the employees feel ill-equipped to handle. Given these characteristics, your strategy for service excellence should include strong team building and substantive and recurring stress-management interventions as well as careful attention to appropriate behavior toward family members who can not only spread the good word about the facility, but who also provide the long-term support system for their loved one.

☐ Chronic Care Settings

Chronic care settings include dialysis units, some rehabilitation settings, radiation therapy, arthritis units, cancer care centers, and the like. In her article "Dealing with Chronic Illness" (*GRIP: Guest Relations in Practice*, 1986 September, 1[4]:1-3), Anna Bloise, senior consultant at the Einstein Consulting Group and a specialist in chronic care, shares her views on what to emphasize in these settings: "The lengthy and repeated health care visits required by chronically ill patients and the resulting intensity of staff involvement magnify the importance of customer relations issues with these populations."

Profile of the Chronic Care Patients and Their Families

Chronic care patients, compared to the general population, are disproportionately composed of elderly people. Staff need to understand the physical and emotional challenges of aging. These patients may develop the following attitudes and problems:

- Adoption of "sick role." Patients with a history of chronic disease may have internalized the "sick" role. They may become dependent, self-focused, and manipulative and want staff to "do" for them even though they still can function for themselves. The challenge to staff is to maximize the patient's independent activity while not dismissing or discounting the patient's need to feel cared for.
- "Bad patient" syndrome. Chronically ill patients may resent feelings of helplessness and dependency and consequently be angry and irritable or complain frequently. Staff can be helped to understand that this "bad patient" syndrome may indicate the patient's need for control. Staff can then direct their efforts toward anticipating needs that the patient cannot meet while maximizing the patient's latitude for choice and control.
- Chronic depression. Chronic depression often goes hand-in-hand with chronic illness. Staff should be aware that they are not responsible for "cheering up" a depressed patient and that superficial niceties may not appropriately address the patient's needs. Patients' negative feelings of anger and sadness should be acknowledged and treated with empathy. Helping patients to identify and

engage in activities that still give pleasure are more effective than the most well-intended "you'll be better soon."

- Loss and past orientation. Chronically ill patients may be acutely aware of functional, sensory, and emotional losses. Absorbed with these feelings of loss, chronically ill patients may dwell on the past more than patients with a better hope of recovery. As with the depressed patient, staff can help the chronically ill by treating them with empathy, listening to recollections of past glories, and focusing on present strengths and abilities.

Families of the chronically ill may be extremely sensitive to the quality of care given the patient, because they feel helpless and guilty at their inability to care for their loved one. As a result, families may be critical of professional care givers. Staff need help to avoid defensive reactions even though the vehemence of the complaint may, from their point of view, exceed the severity of the problem. Letting the family vent frustration and then offering constructive and concrete alternatives for problem solving may diffuse hostility.

Profile of Chronic Care Staff

A customer relations program targeted to chronic care staff needs to address common negative responses to chronically ill patients. Typical staff reactions to their intense relationships with chronic care patients are similar to characteristics of burnout:

- Feelings of failure. Staff may buy into the medical model promoted by doctors that the relapse, deterioration, and death of patients represent the "failure" of the medical system and health care professionals.
- Powerlessness. Staff may feel that their efforts are ineffective or inadequate in making a difference because the patient will not improve. Perceived lack of control is a key factor in burnout.
- Overcompensation. Staff may respond to patient depression by being inappropriately cheerful and ignoring the patient's feelings and concerns.
- The fatigue of intensity. The greater the intensity of interaction with patients, the greater the risk of staff being emotionally drained.
- Withdrawal as defense. Although remaining technically competent, staff may withdraw emotionally to protect their own emotions.
- Resentment of patients. Staff may resent patients' helplessness and respond by stereotyping and treating the patient as an object.

Implications for Customer Relations

Awareness of the unique characteristics of chronic care patients and staff is the first step toward creating targeted customer relations strategies. Staff who remain committed and dedicated, with an ever-renewed sense of challenge and openness to change, are least likely to withdraw from close and caring relationships with patients. Staff need sources of energy and renewal within the job in the form of special programs inside and outside the job, including regular breaks, vacation, continuing education, exercise, and avocations.

To keep staff renewed and open, you must help them to understand that they have certain limitations and opportunities in the chronic care setting:

- Staff should be expected to meet high but not unrealistic expectations. They should be helped to understand clearly what is and isn't reasonably within their control.
- Staff cannot be expected to be all things to a patient who is physically and emotionally needy. They can only be expected to exhibit caring within the basic limitations of their professional role and to seek outside referral for those needs they can't meet.
- Finding out about a patient's life before illness will give staff a sense of the patient as a person before the onset of illness.
- The world of the chronically ill is circumscribed because of functional and sensory losses. Small gestures by caring staff take on great meaning. Excellent customer relations behavior is especially important to chronically ill patients.

Caring and support from other staff and administration are essential. Your strategy for service excellence should provide a support network and open lines of communication. Chronic care staff can and do make a difference in the quality of life of the chronically ill patient. The customer relations strategist should acknowledge the importance of this key employee group by dedicating special training and renewal opportunities to them.

☐ Nursing Homes

The elderly population is growing and so is the number of nursing homes and life-care communities. Because this market segment is becoming increasingly competitive, customer relations strategies that respond to the special needs of the elderly in live-in settings are important from both the humanistic and marketing viewpoints.

Start by breaking through the myths and stereotypes that surround old age. Seniors are not all senile prudes who can never get enough blankets. Train your people to see elderly people as individuals.

Then, consider relationships. Relationships between employees, residents, and family are long term and continuous. Familylike dynamics may take over, producing the emotional mix of love, hostility, helplessness, and guilt. Meanwhile, the family members can be difficult. Perhaps they rarely visit. This situation can frustrate staff who nonetheless are pressed to treat family as customers whether they like them or not. Customer relations strategies must acknowledge the depth and complexity of all these human relationships.

The other important fact in nursing homes is high staff turnover. Your customer relations strategy needs to include strong and frequent orientations of new employees to high standards as well as periodic skill building and supportive help that may lower the traumatic turnover that nursing homes experience.

As is true in psychiatric hospitals and rehabilitation centers, pampering versus pressing for independence is also an issue. What is typically a goal for residents—maximal independence and self-sufficiency—may fly in the face of customer satisfaction. Mrs. Hartwell may get mad when told to "feed yourself because you need to be independent." Once again, explaining why you are refusing the request is extremely important.

On top of these complexities, nursing home residents deserve respect. Customer relations approaches should emphasize behavior that preserves dignity. For example:

- Keeping people covered, and not barging into rooms
- Talking to people as adults; avoiding such condescending remarks as "have you been a good boy since I saw you last" or "hi, sweetheart."
- Speaking in a respectful tone of voice that is not condescending or patronizing
- Interacting in a courteous and polite manner
- Offering choices
- Calling people "Mrs. Simon" instead of "Annie" (unless invited to do otherwise)

In terms of motivating staff for customer relations excellence, employees must be made to understand that they have to overcome the poor public image people seem to have of nursing home care and care givers. Employees can help turn this image around by providing impeccable, caring service to all residents and their loved ones. The result is that they will have increased pride in where they work.

□ Emergency Departments

Having worked with many hospital emergency departments on customer relations, Gail Murphy, consultant with the Einstein Consulting Group, points out that many hospital employees outside of the emergency department see it as a nuisance. Top management has to make all employees and physicians realize that the emergency department is the front door to the hospital. In many cases, more than 50 percent of hospital admissions come through the emergency department door. Efficient, caring treatment there can produce loyal customers for the hospital, people who may under nonemergency conditions have chosen a competitor hospital.

Often, patients who enter through the emergency department doors have to wait hours and hours on stretchers in hallways. They're in luck if they're trauma cases because the staff pay more attention to them while people with lesser ailments seem to get shunted aside. People who need to be admitted to the hospital after their care in the emergency department can wait what seems like an eternity to receive a bed assignment, to get information without pestering the staff, or to be fed during the long hours of waiting for a room.

So what can be done through attention to customer relations?

- Top management needs to communicate to the entire hospital staff that the emergency department is the front door to the hospital and so is important to the hospital's future.
- Confront systems problems that interfere with customer satisfaction. For instance, ensure smooth coordination between the emergency department and ancillary services.
- Emphasize hospitable treatment of the less acute cases. In many emergency departments, staff treat people who are less sick lightly or ignore them. However, these people fume because they feel they are sick and then talk about their poor treatment.
- Identify key staff behaviors that affect patient and family satisfaction: for example, working with upset people, easing long waits, and keeping people informed. Provide training in appropriate skills and give feedback on how well staff are putting these skills into practice.
- Incorporate team building and communication especially between emergency department people and critical care people and between the emergency department staff and the nursing units. Employees throughout the hospital should be helped to view emergency

301

department staff as part of the critical care team instead of outside
of it.
- Help emergency department staff examine the changes in the role
of their department. Work with staff to come to terms with these
changes and to decide together how to make the best of them.
- Focus on teamwork and team building. Obviously, the stress in the
emergency department is great. The focal point of your strategy for
customer relations excellence should be teamwork and the development of mutual support systems that help people cope productively with this hyperstressful environment for the sake of their
patients and themselves.

□ Rural Hospitals

Most rural hospitals start off with a powerful advantage when it
comes to customer relations, and this advantage is smallness. Their
smallness and their typical stature as "the only game in town" have at
least three advantages for service excellence:

- Not only do staff members and physicians tend to have strong ties
to the community, but they also are usually members of the
community. People are not strangers to one another.
- Rural hospitals tend to be low-tech compared with larger and
especially metropolitan hospitals. Rural hospitals have not been
affected by the dehumanization and emphasis on machinery that
have occurred too often in high-tech environments.
- Rural hospitals continue to emphasize the intimacy and friendly
care that have been their tradition.
- Caring and compassion also typically fit the culture of the rural
community. Humanism in the hospital is not threatened by as
much transience, class consciousness, and diversity as is often the
case in urban areas.
- Physicians who practice at rural hospitals typically are loyal to the
hospitals and are long-standing members of the community.

All of these realities make service excellence easier to achieve in
rural hospitals. The rural hospital has fewer employees to reach and so
can reach them more quickly and more often. Physicians tend to see
themselves as less immune to customer relations standards than do
physicians in larger hospitals. Also, customer relations strategies can
be presented as adding strength to a clearly existing tradition of caring
as opposed to starting such a tradition.

Still, rural hospitals face some challenges in customer relations.

The major challenge involves what is reportedly a complacency among staff. Staff members often have a hard time accepting the fact that times have changed and are still changing and that, as a result, more competitive practices have become necessary. The result can be staunch resistance to change.

Another challenge relates to the intimacy among staff and patients. The fact that everyone knows everyone can be both a blessing and a curse. Word travels faster in and about rural hospitals than anywhere else, and professional and friendship roles can become blurred. Thus, rural hospitals have to make sure that staff is constantly reminded about the importance of confidentiality. In fact, sometimes rural people travel miles to a hospital outside their communities just to retain a sense of privacy about their conditions. This tendency is another reason for the continued need to emphasize confidentiality.

Another challenge relates to the fact that rural hospitals seem much like families. Just as families can have internal conflicts and frictions that can be destructive, so can hospitals. Often, a small, rural hospital can best improve its customer relations by focusing on smoothing relationships and interactions among its own employees.

Customer relations and service excellence are just as important to the continued success of rural hospitals as they are to urban hospitals and so cannot be ignored. Rural hospitals need to carefully evaluate their specific environment to determine what they can do to enhance their tradition of caring and compassionate service. Even hospitals that are already good or excellent can always find areas in their organizations that can be improved.

☐ Multicultural Institutions

"All people smile in the same language; and tolerance consists of seeing certain things with your heart, instead of with your eyes."—Baldwin's Brevities

In early 1987, Sandra Kanu Dunn, Ph.D., medical anthropologist and director of Bridges in Health Care in Washington, DC, told the author that "America's 'melting pot' is more like a salad bowl lately, as recent immigrants choose to retain language, ethnic identities, and cultural practices." She points out that the composition of minority groups in the U.S. population is also changing. According to the Center of Health Management Research's *Forecast '87* (Los Angeles: LHS Corporation, 1986), Hispanics will replace Blacks as the largest U.S. minority by 1990. Asian Americans are the fastest growing minority; they will number about 8 million, twice their 1980 numbers.

In health services delivery, the need to strengthen customer relations is especially evident in inner-city areas where recent immigrants tend to cluster. Language barriers, value differences, information gaps, and cultural biases strongly affect the ability of the health care provider to understand patients, their illnesses, and their ability to use the system. As a result, patient satisfaction with services and compliance with medical regimens often suffer.

Other problems minorities have stem from their learned cultural patterns that make some American practices offensive. In her 1986 workshop presentation "Culture-Sensitive Health Care" at the Einstein Training Institute in Philadelphia, Dr. Dunn offers some examples: many Southeast Asian men experience extreme embarrassment if they must undress in front of a woman doctor, and many Southeast Asian women feel inhibited talking to a male psychiatrist. In addition, many people use modern medical services and folk medicines at the same time, with the result that the patient may be endangered. For these and other reasons, customer relations programs in culturally diverse organizations must increase employee sensitivity to the health beliefs and practices common among the cultures that they serve. Such an understanding can overcome the inevitable clash between the culture of the health care provider and the cultural perspectives of patients and families.

In their proposal to the National Health Services Corps in December 1986 (written under the auspices of Miranda Associates, Washington, DC), Dr. Dunn and Noel Chrisman, Ph.D., professor in the College of Nursing at the University of Washington in Seattle, said that culture can be understood in terms of customer relations:

> Culture is more than language or dialect differences, food and dress preferences, or foreign patterns of interpersonal behavior. Culture is a hidden dimension of attitude, world view, and value complexes that underlies people's experience of life.
>
> Life is not experienced the same among peoples of different cultures. The meanings of seemingly similar objects or activities are not necessarily the same across cultures. Compounding the difficulties of this counterintuitive statement about experience differences is the problem of ethnocentrism, the belief that one's own culture's way of life is the only correct one. Ethnocentrism is the key concept in culture-sensitive care. It leads culture members to evaluate the behaviors of members of other cultures as

wrong or bad. When health practitioners do this, they run the risk of not accurately listening to (and therefore assessing) their clients and of devaluing client behaviors and responses to health problems. This is the essence of insensitive and frequently unsafe patient care.

Much of Dr. Dunn's training program aids practitioners to become aware of their own ethnocentrism and to learn how to reduce it in customer care situations. In the newsletter *Guest Relations in Practice* (1986 November, 1[5]:7), Dr. Dunn builds on these premises:

> A culture sensitive approach to service excellence should include "culture brokering." For front-line staff, the idea of brokering is not new. A broker brings together a buyer (the patient) and a seller (the provider). Brokering occurs in intake, screening, financial assistance, and so forth. The broker links the patient with appropriate services and "negotiates" the system for the patient. Although in hospitals, patient representatives, nurses and volunteers may explicitly serve this function, service excellence strategies in multicultural settings should increase the likelihood that every employee sees this kind of brokering as his or her responsibility . . . or at least a function that they can seek on behalf of a befuddled patient.
>
> A culture broker has a specific function . . . to provide and interpret information to both patients and employees. The culture broker is a linking agent and a customer relations coordinator, par excellence. Acting as a linking agent, the culture broker helps to defuse anxiety, decrease the chances of ethnic stereotyping, and increase a health system's ability to handle intercultural situations effectively.

Do you wonder if your hospital should focus attention on intercultural issues? According to Dr. Dunn, the answer is "yes," if the following conditions are present (reprinted with permission of Bridges in Health Care, Washington, DC):

- Patient has:
  —Discomfort with clinical setting
  —Belief in alternative healing cures
  —Minimal English-language proficiency
  —Insistent, repeated use of clinical services
  —Excessive, chronic complaints about services

—Noncompliance with treatment regimens
—Noncompliance with administrative policies
—Fear of asking questions
—Nonbiomedical explanation of illness
- Provider has:
—Mediocentrism: the feeling that Western biomedicine is the only correct and logical method for diagnosis and treatment
—Value differences with patient
—Difficulty coping with the patient's family and friends
—Resentment toward rituals and unique food-preparation requirements
—Fear of AIDS [acquired immune deficiency syndrome]
—Lack of adequate information about the patient
—Favoritism toward certain types of patients
—Bias regarding financial and status differences

Workshops to confront cultural differences and explore the issues described should be conducted with a focus on:

- Contrasts in patient's and provider's cultures
- Interethnic communication
- Multicultural beliefs and their effect on the treatment of illness
- Barriers to seeking care
- Negotiation with patient for compliance with treatment regimens
- Social support for culturally different patients
- Use of culture brokers within the hospital setting
- Provider satisfaction in the face of culture conflict

Sometimes the care givers themselves represent the minority culture and have problems communicating with patients who represent the majority culture in the community. In this case, whether or not formal training programs are offered, supervisors need to ensure that care givers acknowledge cultural issues and develop a repertoire of behaviors that enable care givers to work satisfactorily with patients and their families and friends.

When your front-line employees, such as tray deliverers, transporters, maintenance people, or housekeepers, don't speak the language of the patient, you have a serious customer relations problem. Except for those persons who are gifted in nonverbal signals, employees can't connect with the patient, and so their work, for example, delivering a tray or changing a light bulb, is done in uncomfortable silence.

Employees need specific, concrete help with even the simple situations that recur daily. Other than hiring only multilingual people or running comprehensive language classes, what can you do? Here's a three-step process to help you cope with the problem:

- *Step 1: Identify the phrases that would make the most difference to the patient.* Ask employees for suggestions. For example, tray deliverers could say:
  —"Hello, there. It's nice to see you."
  —"My name is _____, and I'm here to bring you a nice meal."
  —"I'm sorry. I don't understand what you're saying, but I'll find someone to help."
  —"It's nice to see you. I hope you enjoy your meal."
  —"Have a nice day."
- *Step 2: Make sure your people know the appropriate inflection and tone that make the phrases meaningful.* Make sure they understand the importance of eye contact, smiles, and appropriate intonation.
- *Step 3: Require staff to use these or other phrases to make contact with the patient every time they enter the patient's room.* Make this behavior an expectation of each employee's job.

This kind of interaction breaks the ice and the language barrier and enables your employees to warm a patient's hospital stay with human contact.

In summary, says Dr. Dunn, "customer relations programs need to examine structure and procedures from the patient's point of view in order to improve customer relations and increase customer satisfaction. Culture-sensitive health care builds support and enthusiasm for customer relations efforts toward culturally diverse groups by also considering the sociocultural context of the patient's point of view. A training program based on the topics previously discussed adds a highly valued dimension to staff development and guest relations programs" (*GRIP: Guest Relations in Practice,* 1986 November, 1[5]:7).

☐ Final Suggestions

Hospitals vary along a multitude of dimensions. To fashion strategies for service excellence that suit the unique features of your setting, you must beware of these pitfalls:

- *Stereotypes break down.* Don't be too quick to settle on strategies that other settings comparable to yours have used. Slow down and ask yourself whether you see any mitigating factors in your organization that would affect the success of the strategy. The easy answers are dangerous. Have confidence in your own instincts about what will really work in your setting.

- *Stereotypes have a grain of truth.* Although you need to be wary of stereotypes about special settings, you should still tap the experience and resources of organizations similar to yours. One teaching hospital is obviously more like another teaching hospital than it is like a 100-bed rural hospital.
- *Analysis without paralysis is the key.* Given differences between organizations, you need to do careful, thorough groundwork to base your strategy in the reality of your customers' perceptions of your organization and the dynamics and culture of your staff and organization. Skipping initial stock taking is what gets special settings going in a misguided direction.

The issues specific to particular settings that are described in this chapter merely scratch the surface. The point really is that no recipe for customer relations strategies exists. No matter what the overt characteristics of your organization, you need to take a hard look at the particular issues that affect your organization and tailor your strategy to them, no matter what the books or experts or colleagues from another so-called similar organization tell you.

Staying Power: The Follow-Through Challenge

Even after the best of banquets, you have to continue to eat if you want to live. Your strategy for service excellence works the same way. No matter how extravagant or forceful your first helping was, your strategy will starve without a steady diet of maintenance, troubleshooting, and expansion.

In the appendix, you'll find a thorough inventory to help you diagnose your follow-through needs. However, the self-test in figure 19-1 provides a quickie overview. If you answered some "no's" in the self-test, don't feel alone. A comprehensive strategy for service excellence is a long-term, multifaceted effort that you have to strengthen one step at a time. That's the follow-through challenge.

☐ Where to Go Next

Answering the following questions will give you an indication of symptoms that need following up:

- Have you seen slippage in your initial gains?
- Are you disappointed in the behavioral changes you've seen in employees?
- Did your initial strategy leave unfulfilled promises?
- Did your initial efforts generate a backlash of employee resistance to pressures about achieving customer relations excellence?
- Did your initial efforts raise awareness to the point that, now, people are acutely attuned to service dimensions and want to achieve yet higher standards?

Figure 19-1. Self-Test: How "Well" Is Your Strategy for Service Excellence?

Taking Stock. This self-test is designed to give you a quick diagnosis of your follow-through needs. For every "yes" answer, pat yourself on the back for a job well done. For every "no" answer, take a deep breath. You've just found another job that needs doing.

1. Does your strategy for service excellence target patients and their visitors *and* doctors?   Yes   No

2. Have you turned the people in your personnel department into customer relations fanatics, and therefore are job applicants specifically evaluated for customer relations potential?   Yes   No

3. Have your department heads developed written, job-specific customer relations expectations to which they hold employees accountable?   Yes   No

4. Have you fixed the communication snafus (for example, interdepartmental communication and communication from manager to employee or from employee to employee) that used to impede excellent service to customers?   Yes   No

5. Have you convinced your administrative team to keep employees continuously apprised of your organization's competitive position within the local health care marketplace?   Yes   No

6. Does your strategy mobilize every key group, including, for example, housekeeping and tray delivery, so that visitors are surprised by how nice everybody is?   Yes   No

7. An intangible—are your managers genuinely "close" to your customers? Do they talk to them firsthand?   Yes   No

8. Are you involving your doctors in a strategy to improve their own behavior toward patients and employees?   Yes   No

9. Have you weaned employees from using stress as an excuse for mediocrity?   Yes   No

10. Have you given special attention to building the job-specific skills of groups with the most patient contact, for example, admissions personnel, patient representatives, transporters, nurses?   Yes   No
(continued)

Figure 19-1. *(continued)*

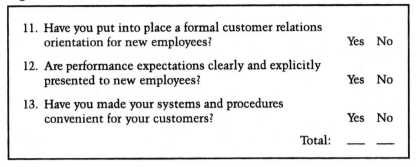

11. Have you put into place a formal customer relations orientation for new employees? Yes No

12. Are performance expectations clearly and explicitly presented to new employees? Yes No

13. Have you made your systems and procedures convenient for your customers? Yes No

Total: __ __

If you're an old-timer at customer relations, these questions may get you thinking about all the things you've done right and all the things you've done wrong in your strategy so far. If you're a novice, you may be fretting about all the things you wish you had done already. However, bemoaning the past makes no sense.

What distinguishes a successful strategy for service excellence from an unsuccessful one is not why it came into being (for the right or wrong reasons, narrow or enlightened) and not what kind of program you put in place and whether it proved to be on target or off base. *What distinguishes a successful customer relations strategy from an unsuccessful one is not its past, but its future.*

So, how do you go about finding out which aspects of your strategy are working and which are not? And how do you plan your next steps?

Start with an audit. Collect information from your customers outside and inside the hospital by using focus groups, surveys, face-to-face interviews, user-friendly committees, and the like. Get your key people together, ideally in a retreat setting, to process your customer relations results. Have a strong facilitator on hand who can summarize, focus, and define priorities. Typically, top management and task force members should participate. You can structure these retreats as follows:

- Take stock of your past customer relations efforts, their strengths and weaknesses. Use the 10 pillars of customer relations excellence (chapter 4 and part II of this book) to aid your analysis.
- Compare your results so far with your original goals and hopes. Use the service matrix (figure 7-7) to aid your analysis.
- Identify and tackle issues related to leadership of and responsibility for your strategy for service excellence.
- Examine alternative strategies for strengthening, troubleshooting, and following through on your efforts.
- Develop a sequenced, achievable action plan for follow-through.

- Develop an implementation strategy that spells out what, when, and by whom.

A priority like customer relations excellence deserves a long-term strategic plan. The results of such a planning retreat can help your key people build just the blueprint or game plan that they need to keep your strategy on course.

☐ Document the Need for Follow-Through

Of course, the implementation of a follow-through strategy takes resources and support. Experience suggests that the in-house people who direct customer relations strategies need to build a strong case for continued efforts. Too often, top management makes an up-front commitment to customer relations but expects that after an initial show of financial and moral support, they can channel the organization's resources elsewhere. To make sure the powers-that-be won't cop out, you need an approach for lobbying for the sustenance your strategy needs. Here are nine steps involved in building a strong, assertive case for attention and support for follow-through:

- Figure out what your strategy needs to entail. What resources and support do you need or want in order to accomplish your plan?
- Identify your real reasons for believing that these resources and support are necessary.
- Identify the key people or groups whose support you need in order to make your plan a reality.
- Anticipate all the reasons why key people or groups in your organization may resist giving you what you need.
- Spell out in sufficient detail all the ways the key people in your organization would benefit from supporting the plan you've laid out. Specifically, spell out in advance exactly how each of the following individuals and groups will benefit:
  —You
  —Your staff
  —Your department
  —Physicians
  —The administration
  —Your boss in particular
  —The organization
  —Patients and visitors
  —Employees
- Develop in detail the costs of the effort and the risks involved.

Consider financial costs, people costs, emotional costs, time, aggravation, and so forth. You have to show you've thought of everything and aren't proceeding blindly or naively.

- Now put it all together. Make an articulate, convincing case that your organization cannot *thrive* without this well-considered follow-through strategy. Show your understanding of the costs as well as the benefits. Explain why the potential benefits outweigh the costs.

- Propose desired and rational timing for a decision and for the plan's implementation. If you build a strong case for a timely decision, you have a reason for persistently asking for the verdict. This persistence gets the attention of higher-ups, who could as easily table this priority plan if they feel no pressure.

- Remain confident and assertive. Expect that those with authority will see the excellent sense you're making and back the plan. If you don't receive the support you're seeking, act surprised and persist. Don't give up easily. If you get a "no" and you're convinced the organization is making a big mistake, start over. Find support in your committee. Cultivate influential opinion leaders. Go through the whole process again. Try as many times as is necessary to prove your point. If you really believe in your cause and in your plan and in yourself, then you've really got a case.

☐ Follow-Through Options

First of all, figure out which service dimensions and which customer groups you want to address most immediately. Use the customer service matrix (figure 7-7) to help you focus. Then, consider the 10 pillars of customer relations excellence, which are discussed briefly in chapter 4 and more fully in part II. Identify achievements and gaps. Gaps are ripe areas for follow-through activities. The following eight standard directions are ones that ambitious organizations pursue in customer relations follow-through:

- *From people skills to systems.* So many hospitals start by focusing on employee behavior toward customers. This focus is, after all, a good first step in building a service orientation among employees. However, after people are aware and new, higher behavioral expectations infuse the organization's policies and practices, people tend to find that their ability to extend themselves to the organization's customers is hampered by systems that oppress everyone. Long waits, hard-to-decipher forms, misplaced charts, and duplicate lab testing, for example, are all a function of problematic systems that make it difficult for even the best people to show compassion and care day after day. According to Katie Buckley of the Einstein Consulting Group, "Focusing exclusively on people skills despite harrowing systems problems is like having ice cream dipped in chocolate. As you begin to savor it, the inside melts and the structure collapses." For many organizations, an overt attack on systems problems that have plagued the organization for years is perfect for follow-through.

- *From people skills to service management.* Once a service orientation is uppermost in people's minds, you can begin to see that many departments are not structured as service delivery systems and that their managers are not thinking like managers of service businesses. The transition to service management is another important direction for follow-through. During this transition, top and middle management literally need to be retrained (or replaced) to run their domains as functional departments that provide service to customers and to remember that often those customers are fellow departments, not just patients. Service management involves systems for staying in touch with all customers; staying competitive in the services provided; letting customer needs, not the providers' needs, dictate policy and procedure; restructuring hours and jobs to remove access barriers; pinpointing responsibility so it is not allowed to ricochet from person to person and place to place; increasing the time it takes to respond to people's needs and make decisions; standardizing customer service procedures; building in strong, ongoing training for personnel so that they manage moments of truth and customer pressure points well; and increasing decisive steps to improve the department's services and user friendliness at minimal cost to the organization. This service-management approach takes substantive, long-term training because few health care managers matured in systems that demanded this kind of management performance. Allan Geller, consultant with the Einstein Consulting Group, summarizes the training needs of the "new-age middle manager in health care." Managers must be trained to:
  —Move from passive to active response.
  —Move from a focus on turf protection to a focus on integrated service orientation.
  —Become active problem solvers.
  —Behave in entrepreneurial ways to sharpen the functioning of areas of responsibility.
  —Think about what's good for the organization and not just about what's good for a specific department.
  —Exercise managerial courage, require conformity to high stan-

dards, hold people accountable, and fire employees if necessary.
—Build strong teams of believers in the organization.
—Get off the dime or leave.

- *Custom strategies for specific customer groups.* Take physicians for instance. Many customer relations programs have done nothing to involve the doctors. A follow-through strategy may involve making the tough decision necessary to develop and institute a meaningful physician strategy, whether the strategy treats the doctors as customers who are right even when they're wrong or as care givers who are expected to conform to the standards of behavior that apply to the organization's entire work force.

- *Genuine revamping of internal systems for input, problem solving, and communication.* Building a responsive, self-correcting system is what is important. Frequently this action entails more administrative attention to employee needs and concerns and more employee participation in problem solving. Facilitating this change is not easy. It takes a renewed commitment on the part of top management to focus attention on the inside of the organization—on the employee as customer—and to be less single-mindedly focused on external forces.

- *Beyond lip service from top management.* Top management can do only so much to infuse the organization and its people with service excellence and a customer orientation. Service excellence takes time and dedicated attention. Often, it also requires personal changes on the part of managers, both top management and supervisors. For example, they may need to wander around more, improve social skills, or make a commitment to call one customer per day. The appropriate management focus is the single most efficient customer relations intervention. Once top managers act visionary, that is, align themselves toward service excellence, they do many things automatically that move people and the organization forward.

- *Employee-as-customer strategies.* Bold hospitals are pursuing the employee as customer as the thrust for their follow-through strategy. These hospitals have learned that employees just don't sell their organizations unless they believe in it, have confidence in it, and know the ins and outs of the services provided in it. Also, happy employees make happy patients, and as a result, employees' basic needs merit attention. When you treat employees as customers, you rethink perks, raises, cutbacks, and rituals that pull together the organizational family. You conduct in-house information campaigns so that employees know the organization's news before the public hears it. You teach employees basic sales skills, and you take pains to solicit and address employee concerns and needs. Two

315

beliefs underlie these activities: *the committed employee sells your organization, and customer relations is merely the mirror image of employee relations.*

- *Caring for the care giver.* In these days of escalating pressures on the care givers, an entirely new angle for follow-through has to do with professional renewal, or caring for the care giver. The underlying premise is that the care giver who works happy is more successful with the customer and more positive about the organization. A professional renewal approach to follow-through does not apply yet more pressure on already tired people to be nicer to the customer. Instead, it helps people reorganize their approach to work so that they derive satisfactions from it. The result is renewed energy and commitment to the job and to your organization's customers.
- *Conscientious, targeted skill building.* The other follow-through theme that advances your people from good to excellent in customer relations behavior is skill building through training. Ideally, this approach entails job-specific skill building designed to identify in each person's specific position the missed opportunities that mark the distance between mediocrity and excellence. A training agenda that reaches one job-specific group after another is pay dirt for customer relations follow-through.

☐ An Annual Plan

The right combination of follow-through activities depends on your organization's progress and needs. Ideally, you will, after a planning retreat, develop at least a one-year game plan that has a pattern to it. If you have a pattern, you are less likely to exhaust yourself endlessly considering the multitude of possibilities and just commit yourself to making your plan a reality, step by step.

Some hospitals even develop a format for an annual plan. Then, each year, they plug in the specifics. Following is one hospital's blueprint for follow-through:

- Service excellence planning retreat
- Annual refresher for all employees
- Management renewal
- Quarterly customer relations articles for house publication
- Annual poster contest with rotating posters
- Two contests per year for solving particular service improvement problems
- Team-building intervention with troubled departments

- Professional renewal workshop series for particularly burned-out groups
- Ongoing follow-through committees with their own action plans:
  —User-friendly committee
  —Reward and recognition
  —Fun events
  —Management effectiveness
  —Employee relations
  —Physician relations
- A training series for middle managers and supervisors
- A training series for job-specific employee groups
- An annual theatrical event that pokes fun and revives a customer orientation

☐ Four Necessary Functions in Follow-Through

Unfortunately, no formula exists for follow-through. As is true with any challenging organizational priority, progress over the long haul takes periodic stock taking, planning, and implementation and then more stock taking, planning, and implementation in an endless cyclical process.

However, one thing is clear. The people involved in advancing your strategy need to be committed and visionary. They also need to fulfill four necessary functions throughout the life of your strategy. Borrowing the four hats of the creative person developed by Roger Von Oech in *A Kick in the Seat of the Pants*, (New York City: Perennial Library, Harper & Row, 1986), your service excellence team needs to serve as explorers, judges, artists, and warriors in order to press your strategy forward:

- *Be the explorer.* Your team needs to collect information and scrutinize your results along the way with an eye to understanding the dynamics that are causing success or disappointment. Look for relationships, breakdowns, barriers, dips, and swings. Look to other industries to see how they stay in touch with their customers and meet their needs. Look at how plumbers solve those difficult systems problems. Your follow-through plans will be most appropriate if they are grounded in a knowledge of the territory.
- *Be the artist.* Having gathered all this information and knowing your problems and weaknesses, your team needs to draw into your strategic process creative people who can help you craft solutions that create the textures, colors, and forms to suit your people, culture, and problems. The artist, remember, chips away at the

317

sculpture to create the work of art. Remove the constraints to people's thinking and encourage the freewheeling creativity that may just help your people stride or even leapfrog forward.

- *Be the judge.* Your team needs to be discerning and strategic and to courageously acknowledge what is working and what is not and pick and choose what will enhance your strategy and its results. Letting problems slip by year after year, letting people who drag down your organization's image do so year after year, adopting strategy ideas that are weak or unjustifiably costly or difficult, these actions reveal an unwillingness to judge and take action for the sake of your vision of service excellence.

- *Be the warrior.* The warrior has stamina. Perhaps it's all that adrenalin pumping. The warrior may be obsessed with the objective. The warrior will ramrod through and over obstacles to get to the objective. Your team needs to be the warrior for service excellence. You and your team need to lobby, assert yourselves, advocate, and persist for what you know needs to happen.

☐ A Prediction

Where is all this going? You strategize, you follow through, you devote energy and resources to service excellence, and you wear yourself out doing it.

The only reason that hospitals are paying so much attention to the pursuit of service excellence is that hospitals are facing heightened consumer expectations that are demanding a conversion to service-oriented cultures. Eventually, hospitals will have weathered the storm of this far-reaching cultural change. They will exude a strong service orientation that drives their behavior, systems, and decisions. When hospitals reach this point, customer relations will require dramatically less deliberate attention because it will be an everyday management priority, a habit. It will be in every manager's bloodstream.

However, until that utopia arrives, and to sustain it once it does, you have to do all you can to help your organization achieve the objective of service excellence for the sake of patients and their family and friends and for the sake of employees and physicians whose job satisfaction, spirit, and effectiveness depend so much on the organization's service integrity. Hopefully, this book will spur you and your organization forward.

Customer Relations Needs Inventory and Scoring Manual

□ Customer Relations Needs Inventory

Directions. This needs inventory helps you diagnose the strengths and weaknesses in your organization's customer relations strategy. Think about your organization right now. Consider each statement on this survey, and check "yes" or "no" for each item as it applies to your organization. If only part of the statement is true for your organization, check "no." Force yourself to choose the best answer, even if you'd prefer to answer "somewhat" or "maybe."

A. Management Philosophy and Commitment

1. Your administrative team communicates often about the mission and values underlying your priority of service excellence.   Yes   No

2. Your administrative teams makes a deliberate effort to be visible and available to all levels of staff and seeks out opportunities to become actively involved in the effort for service excellence.   Yes   No

3. Recognizing the power of management as role models, your administrative team sets clear and high standards of behavior for themselves and for their subordinates.   Yes   No

4. When needed, your administrative team volunteers to use their clout to ensure cooperation with every facet of your strategy for service excellence.   Yes   No

5. Even when the news is bad or uncomfortable to discuss, your administrative team tells employees the truth about issues that affect customer relations goals (for example, layoffs, downsizing, patient survey results, and the like).   Yes   No

6. Your administrative team has made a commitment to becoming more service oriented by responding to the needs of key user groups.   Yes   No

TOTAL   ____   ____

B. Accountability

1. Courteous, respectful, and compassionate behavior toward patients and other customers is a *requirement* in your organization, not an option.   Yes   No

2. Clear behavioral expectations that describe customer relations behavior in specific terms have been written for all employees.   Yes   No

3. Managers and supervisors hold employees accountable for their behavior toward hospital customers, and they confront problem employees when such employees hurt the hospital's image.   Yes   No

4. At your hospital, managers and supervisors are encouraged to coach, discipline, and eventually terminate employees who persist in their failure to meet high standards for service excellence.   Yes   No

5. Department heads and supervisors who are technically competent but are negative in their interpersonal skills toward employees and hospital customers are under pressure to meet customer relations standards.   Yes   No

6. The atmosphere in your organization makes it impossible any longer for rude and belligerent employees to remain secure and accepted year after year.   Yes   No

7. Your department heads and supervisors have established and communicated clear, job-specific expectations to the people they supervise.   Yes   No

8. Your administrators have communicated clear expectations to the people they supervise.   Yes   No

9. Specific customer relations responsibilities are built into job descriptions.   Yes   No

10. Your hiring practices include specific techniques for screening applicants for customer relations instincts and skills.   Yes   No

11. Customer relations behavior has a prominent place in your performance appraisal process.   Yes   No

12. Your new employee orientation emphasizes the importance you place on customer satisfaction and communicates the specific behavior expected of every employee to achieve customer satisfaction.   Yes   No

TOTAL   ____   ____

C. Input and Evaluation

1. You have systems in place to assess visitor satisfaction with your staff and services.   Yes   No

2. You have systems in place to assess patient satisfaction with your staff and services.   Yes   No

3. You have systems in place to tap physician satisfaction with your staff and services.   Yes   No

4. You have systems in place to tap employee satisfaction with their coworkers, managers, work environment, and hospital systems.   Yes   No

5. You're confident that your evaluation return rate is high enough to give you an accurate representation.   Yes   No

6. You ask focused customer relations questions; the information you get from your evaluation strategies is specific and clear enough to accurately tell you how you're doing with customer relations.   Yes   No

TOTAL   _____   _____

D. Problem Solving and Complaint Management

1. When patients have a complaint or concern, they know whom to call.   Yes   No

2. You have a clear, smooth-running system for handling patient complaints and needs.   Yes   No

3. You have a system for communicating back to patients any actions taken as a result of their complaints or requests.   Yes   No

4. When visitors have a complaint or concern, they know whom to call.   Yes   No

5. You have a clear, smooth-running system for handling visitor complaints and needs.   Yes   No

6. You have a system for communicating back to visitors any actions taken as a result of their complaints or requests.   Yes   No

7. When physicians have a complaint or concern, they know whom to call.   Yes   No

8. You have a clear, smooth-running system for handling physician complaints and needs.   Yes   No

9. You have a system for communicating back to physicians any actions taken as a result of their complaints or requests.   Yes   No

10. When employees have complaints or suggestions, they know specific channels for expressing them.   Yes   No

11. Your administration and middle managers usually respond to employee complaints and concerns, even if they don't act on them.   Yes   No

12. Your administration is generally perceived as open to employee complaints and suggestions.   Yes   No

                                    TOTAL   ____   ____

E. Downward Communication
1. Your employees at all levels are regularly informed about your hospital's financial situation and competitive position.   Yes   No

2. You have a system for updating your employees on the economic challenges ahead for your organization so that they know how you're doing and what you're doing to succeed.   Yes   No

3. Your employees are well informed about decisions made by top management and about the real reasons for those decisions.   Yes   No

4. Your administrators and department heads share information openly with employees, especially during hard times.   Yes   No

5. You regularly use a variety of methods for communicating with staff (for example, memos, meetings, newsletters, "town meetings").   Yes   No

6. Your administrators and managers encourage questions and requests for information and respond quickly to these even if they don't have a clear or final answer yet.   Yes   No

                                    TOTAL   ____   ____

F. Staff Development and Training
1. Your organization offers ongoing training to upgrade the customer relations skills of all employees, from administrators to front-line employees.   Yes   No

2. You assess the training needs of your staff and tailor training programs to meet their real needs.   Yes   No

3. You provide the support needed so employees can and do attend training programs. Yes No

4. You offer professional renewal programs to help your nurses and others handle the stress, pressure, and burnout felt by many these days. Yes No

5. You have strategies for team building so that problems within groups and between groups are not ignored. Yes No

6. In all of your training programs, you reinforce the goals of your customer relations effort and make it clear that the training is offered to help employees meet these goals. Yes No

TOTAL ____ ____

G. Physician Involvement
1. You have a well-planned strategy for continued physician involvement because you view the physician as customer and team member. Yes No

2. You have methods for involving physicians in planning their own involvement. Yes No

3. Your physicians are aware of your organization's priority on customer relations. Yes No

4. Your physicians see themselves as an important part of your customer relations strategy. Yes No

5. You've made physicians aware of the specific behavioral expectations that constitute positive customer relations. Yes No

6. When a physician violates your customer relations standards, that physician is confronted in a constructive way. Yes No

TOTAL ____ ____

H. Reward and Recognition
1. Your organization has working systems for recognizing employees who are wonderful to customers. Yes No

2. Your reward and recognition systems reinforce the behavior patterns expected in your customer relations strategy. Yes   No

3. Your reward and recognition systems allow for the acknowledgment of groups, departments, and individuals on all levels. Yes   No

4. Your reward and recognition systems acknowledge many people who are customer relations superstars, not just a select few. Yes   No

5. Your department heads develop and use reward and recognition systems within their own departments, in addition to organizationwide systems. Yes   No

6. Your employees value your reward and recognition systems; they strive to be selected and acknowledged. Yes   No

TOTAL   ____ ____

I. Employee as Customer

1. Your employees feel appreciated and valued. Yes   No

2. Your administration realizes that happy employees make patients happy. Yes   No

3. You have a system for gathering and addressing the needs of your employees. Yes   No

4. You invite employee participation before making changes that will affect them. Yes   No

5. You know you have to sell your employees on your services and goals before you can expect them to sell these to your external customers. Yes   No

6. You pay explicit attention to the need for employees to see their coworkers as customers who deserve excellent service. Yes   No

TOTAL   ____ ____

J. Reminders, Refreshers, Attention Grabbers

1. You generate periodic visual reminders that reinforce customer relations messages (for example, posters, T-shirts, buttons).   Yes   No

2. Your house publications carry features on customer relations issues, events, and accomplishments.   Yes   No

3. You sponsor contests and events focusing on customer relations themes to keep people energized.   Yes   No

4. You conduct periodic organizationwide workshops that revive awareness and commitment.   Yes   No

5. Your employees see that your customer relations commitment is ongoing, not a flash-in-the-pan.   Yes   No

6. Whether employees have been with you for 20 years or 1 year, they're well aware of your customer relations commitment.   Yes   No

TOTAL   ___   ___

☐ Scoring Manual

How To Score

1. Make sure you've responded to every item.
2. Count the number of "yes" answers for each section and write the total for each at the end of that section.
3. Now transfer the totals for each section to the block below in the column that reads "Total."

	Section	Total	X	Factor	=	Score
Management philosophy and commitment	A	[ ]	X	2	=	[ ]
Accountability	B	[ ]	X	1	=	[ ]
Input and evaluation	C	[ ]	X	2	=	[ ]
Problem solving and complaint management	D	[ ]	X	1	=	[ ]
Downward communication	E	[ ]	X	2	=	[ ]
Staff development and training	F	[ ]	X	2	=	[ ]
Physician involvement	G	[ ]	X	2	=	[ ]
Reward and recognition	H	[ ]	X	2	=	[ ]
Employee as customer	I	[ ]	X	2	=	[ ]
Reminders, refreshers, attention grabbers	J	[ ]	X	2	=	[ ]

4. Now multiply each total above by the factor next to it, and write the answer in the column on the right.
5. Now look at the next section to see how your scores should be interpreted.

How to Interpret Your Score

Your score indicates your degree of success in each category. The highest score possible for each category is 12. The higher the number, the better. Lower numbers reflect gaps or weaknesses in your strategy. To learn from these, go back and analyze the specific items that deflated your score, because these areas reveal promising directions for follow-up.

A. Management Philosophy and Commitment

Customer relations strategies need to be driven specifically by an explicit value on customer relations excellence. The higher your score, the more your top management shows a commitment to these values. The lower your score, the more you need to slow down and take a hard look at what your top management needs to do to strive to exemplify and communicate customer relations values and commitment.

B. Accountability

Does your customer relations strategy have "teeth"? Lower scores here indicate a weak foundation. Employees may know about the value your organization places on customer relations, but without accountability mechanisms, you can't expect lasting results. Consider these options:

- Institute mandatory customer relations job requirements in behavioral terms. Build these requirements into policies, job descriptions, new employee orientations, hiring practices, performance appraisals, and disciplinary procedures.
- Arrange for focused training of administrators, middle managers, and supervisors on their role in achieving customer relations excellence. Include skills in being a role model, setting and communicating job-specific expectations, and reinforcing and enforcing high standards.

C. Input and Evaluation

You need to stay close to your customers and the people who make your organization tick. Do you have ongoing, effective methods for evaluating the satisfaction of patients, visitors, physicians, and employees? A perfect score means you not only have systems for evaluating satisfaction, but you also receive a high enough return and feel confident that your information paints an accurate picture. If your score is less than perfect, consider broadening your evaluation strategies to get input from all customer groups or fine-tune your strategies so more people respond to questions that measure how you're doing in customer relations.

D. Problem Solving and Complaint Management

What happens with the data you gather from patients, visitors, physicians, and employees? Unless you funnel it into problem-solving processes or into the hands of people with the power to listen and act, you're wasting a precious opportunity to improve your organization and tackle the problems that dissatisfy your customers.

You also make people angry. After all, they realize that although asked what they think, no one intends to do anything about it. A lower score means you need to beef up systems for problem solving and complaint gathering, handling, and communicating back to those who complained.

E. Downward Communication
Employee morale is defeated more by no news than by bad news. Employees will be committed to your organization only if management keeps them informed about how the organization is doing, what people are doing, and why decisions are made or not made. If your score is high, congratulations. You have strong systems for downward communication that keep people informed. If your score is low, you need to build new systems or strengthen existing systems for sharing information.

F. Staff Development and Training
The people skills that constitute excellent customer relations are not easy. Impressing your customers with your compassionate, responsive, and respectful treatment is not easy. It takes skill. Lower scores in this area suggest the need for skill-building programs and other employee development strategies. Make sure your employee development strategies include assessing skills so you're providing what people really need most in their specific jobs.

G. Physician Involvement
If physicians are not involved in your strategy for service excellence, then your employees are probably angry. Also, physicians are care givers and part of the team, so how can you ignore them? Lower scores in this area indicate a need to develop or strengthen your physician strategy. The shape of it depends on the role and structure of your physician groups (for example, voluntary, full-time staff, residents, students, a combination, and so forth). Consider the following:

- Physician focus groups to decide how best to reach physicians.
- Briefings or workshops for physicians about your overall strategy and how physicians can help; behavioral expectations for physicians

H. Reward and Recognition
As part of your strategy for service excellence, you need to acknowledge and reward those staff members who deserve it, in other words, those persons who have distinguished themselves by their exemplary energy, behavior, and sense of commitment. If you scored low on this component, you need to develop and implement systems for reinforc-

ing the behaviors you value among individuals, groups, and departments.

I. Employee as Customer
If your employees are demoralized or feel unappreciated and devalued in your environment, they are hardly able or likely to win patients and other customers for your organization. To sustain a satisfied and productive work force, you have to make your workplace a nourishing place to work. The lower your score, the more you need to develop strategies for treating your employees as customers and for encouraging your employees to treat one another as customers.

J. Reminders, Refreshers, Attention Grabbers
Unless you take action to remind people of your customer relations priority and refresh their minds, mind sets, and approaches, awareness fades. Consider consciously instituting methods that trigger attention to customer relations. Well-intentioned people with their hearts in the right place just may not be thinking about customer relations. If you scored low in this area, consider the many options for visual reminders, energizers, and refresher programs to rejuvenate customer relations with your employees.

Selected Bibliography

Albrecht, Karl, and Zemke, Ron. *Service America: Doing Business in the New Economy.* Homewood, IL: Dow Jones-Irwin, 1985.

Bloch, Thomas M., Upah, Gregory, and Zeithaml, Valarie. *Services Marketing in a Changing Environment.* Chicago, IL: American Marketing Association, Proceedings Series, 1985.

Califano, Joseph A., Jr. *America's Healthcare Revolution: Who Lives! Who Dies! Who Pays!* New York City: Random House, 1986.

Coile, Russell C., Jr. *The New Hospital: Future Strategies for a Changing Industry.* Rockville, MD: Aspen Publishing, 1986.

Deal, Terrence E., and Kennedy, Allan A. *Corporate Cultures: The Rites and Rituals of Corporate Life.* Reading, MA: Addison-Wesley Publishing Co., 1982.

Deal, Terrance E., Kennedy, Allan A., and Spiegel, Arthur H. III. How to create an outstanding hospital culture. *Hospital Forum.* 1983 Jan.-Feb. 26(1):21-34.

Friedman, Emily. What do consumers really want? *Healthcare Forum.* 1986 May-June. 29(3):19-24.

Fritz, Rita L. Developing a consumer-driven hospital: four fatal flaws. *Healthcare Forum.* 1986 May-June. 29(3):39-40.

George, William R., and Compton, Fran. How to initiate a marketing perspective in a health services organization. *Journal of Health Care Marketing.* 1985 Winter. 5(1):29-37.

Goldsmith, Martin, and Leebov, Wendy. Strengthening the hospital's marketing position through training. *Healthcare Management Review.* 1986 Spring. 11(2):83-93.

Hickman, Craig, and Silva, Michael. *Creating Excellence.* New York City: New American Library, 1984.

Jenna, Judith K. Toward the patient-driven hospital. *Healthcare Forum.* 1986 May-June. 29(3):8-18.

Kotler, Philip, and Clarke, Roberta N. Creating the responsive organization. *Healthcare Forum.* 1986 May-June. 29(3):27-36.

Kurman, Marsha. Customer relations: the personnel angle. *Personnel.* 1987 Sept. 64(9):38-40.

Leebov, Wendy, and Goldsmith, Martin. How to create a more consumer-oriented work force. *Personnel Administrator.* 1984 Oct. 29(10):99-109.

_____. Does your customer relations program have what it takes? *The Hospital Manager.* 1985 Jan.-Feb. 15(1):4-6.

Leebov, Wendy, and Kurman, Marsha. Dealing with resistance to guest relations. *Hospital Manager.* 1986 May-June. 16(3):4.

Levitt, Theodore. *The Marketing Imagination.* New York City: MacMillan, Inc., The Free Press, 1983.

Peters, Thomas J. Common courtesy: the ultimate barrier to entry. *Hospital Forum.* 1984 Jan.-Feb. 27(1):10-16.

Peters, Thomas J., and Austin, Nancy K. *A Passion for Excellence: The Leadership Difference.* New York City: Random House, 1985.

Peters, Thomas J., and Waterman, Robert H., Jr. *In Search of Excellence.* New York City: Harper and Row, Inc., 1982.

Van Den Haag, Ernest. How to make hospitals hospitable. *Fortune.* 1982 May 17. 105(10):123-27.

Venkatesan, M., Schmalensee, Diane M., and Marshall, Claudia. *Creativity in Services Marketing.* San Francisco, CA: American Marketing Association, Proceedings Series, 1985.

Waterman, Robert H., Jr. *The Renewal Factor.* New York City: Bantam Books, 1987.

0-595-28367-5